O8-CCO-919

Antithrombotic Therapy

Second Edition

Richard C. Becker, MD

Professor of Medicine
Director, Cardiovascular Thrombosis
Research Center
Director, Coronary Care Unit
Director, Anticoagulation Services
University of Massachusetts
Medical School

Dan J. Fintel, MD

Associate Professor of Medicine
Northwestern University School of Medicine
Director of Coronary Care Unit
Northwestern Memorial Hospital

David Green, MD, PhD

Professor of Medicine
Director of Atherosclerosis Program
Northwestern University School of Medicine
Director of Northwestern Hemophilia Center
Northwestern Memorial Hospital

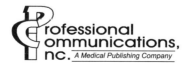

Professional
Communications,
Inc. *A Medical Publishing Company*

Published by
Professional Communications, Inc.

Marketing Office:	*Editorial Office:*
400 Center Bay Drive	PO Box 10
West Islip, NY 11795	Caddo, OK 74729-0010
(t) 631/661-2852	(t) 580/367-9838
(f) 631/661-2167	(f) 580/367-9989

For orders, please call
1-800-337-9838

or visit our website
www.pcibooks.com

ISBN: 1-884735-68-1

Printed in the United States of America

DISCLAIMER
The opinions expressed in this publication reflect those of the authors. However, the authors make no warranty regarding the contents of the publication. The protocols described herein are general and may not apply to a specific patient. Any product mentioned in this publication should be taken in accordance with the prescribing information provided by the manufacturer.

This text is printed on recycled paper.

DEDICATION

Dedicated to the investigation and optimal care of patients with atherothrombosis involving the cardiovascular, peripheral vascular, and cerebrovascular systems.

ACKNOWLEDGMENT

We graciously acknowledge the tireless and unconditional dedication of physicians, nurses, and support staff at Northwestern Memorial Hospital and the UMASS-Memorial Medical Center.

TABLE OF CONTENTS

v

TABLES

FIGURES

1

Role of Clotting Factors and Fibrinolysis in Thrombus Formation

Introduction

The fluidity of the blood is maintained by a balance of procoagulants and anticoagulants. Activation of coagulation initially tips the balance in favor of the procoagulants, but as these proteins become activated they not only increase the clotting ability of the blood but also participate in the activation of the anticoagulant proteins, serving to restore the hemostatic balance. Thus coagulation is a dynamic process, with thrombin generation and inhibition, and fibrin formation and fibrin lysis, all occurring in varying degrees at any given moment.

Procoagulant and anticoagulant factors, their plasma concentrations, and half-lives are listed in Table 1.1.[1]

Initiation of Thrombosis

The initiating event in blood coagulation is injury to the vessel wall. Monocytes, neutrophils, and macrophages are attracted to the site of injury and elaborate tissue factor, an integral membrane glycolipoprotein of 50 kd.[2] To express its procoagulant activity, tissue factor must be anchored to a phospholipid membrane; it then forms a complex with factor VII and activated factor VII (VIIa), which constitutes about 1% of the circulating factor VII[3] (Figure 1.1). The binding of tissue factor to VIIa produces a powerful procoagulant complex, which cleaves its substrates, factor IX and factor X. With the cleavage of factor X to its active form, factor Xa, anticoagulant mechanisms are set into motion. Tissue factor pathway inhibitor (TFPI) is a 32 kd protein that is a potent protease inhibitor that binds to and inactivates Xa. Furthermore, the TFPI-Xa complex inhibits the tissue factor-VIIa complex.

TABLE 1.1 — PROCOAGULANT AND ANTICOAGULANT FACTORS

Protein	Concentration (nM)	$t_{\frac{1}{2}}$ (days)
Fibrinogen	7000	3 to 5
Prothrombin	1400	2.5
Factor V	20	0.5
Factor VII	10	0.25
Factor VIII	0.7	0.5
Factor IX	90	1
Factor X	170	1.25
Factor XI	30	3
Factor XIII	30	9
TFPI	2.5	*
Protein C	60	0.25
Protein S	300	1.75
Antithrombin	2400	3

Abbreviations: $t_{\frac{1}{2}}$, half-life; TFPI, tissue factor pathway inhibitor.

* 80 minutes in animals.

Mann KG, et al. In: *Hematology.* 5th ed. New York, NY: McGraw-Hill Inc; 1995:1206.

Factor IXa may be formed from factor IX by the contact activation system, which consists of factor XII, high molecular weight kininogen (HMWK), prekallikrein (PK), and factor XI.[4-6]

Thrombin is formed in trace amounts by the action of Xa on prothrombin (right half of Figure 1.1). Thrombin also activates factors V (Va) and VIII (VIIIa), which serve as cofactors for Xa and IXa, respectively. A complex forming on the surface of activated platelets consisting of IXa, VIIIa, and calcium ions activates factor X (Xa); it is termed the tenase complex. The Xa generated that escapes TFPI

FIGURE 1.1 — ACTIVATION OF BLOOD COAGULATION

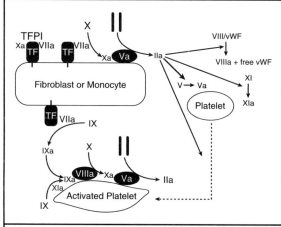

Tissue factor (TF), presented by fibroblasts or monocytes, binds factor VIIa. While most of the TF-VIIa complex is inactivated by factor Xa-tissue factor pathway inhibitor (TFPI), TF-VIIa escaping inactivation converts factor X to factor Xa. Factor Xa along with factor Va activates prothrombin (II) to thrombin (IIa), which in turn activates platelets, converts factor V to Va, factor XI to XIa, and factor VIII to VIIIa after factor VIII dissociates from von Willebrand's factor (vWF). The TF-VIIa complex also activates factor IX to IXa, which, along with VIIIa on the activated platelet surface, converts X to Xa. Factor Xa with Va activates II to thrombin (IIa). XIa on the activated platelet surface also activates IX to IXa.

Roberts HR, et al. *Haemophilia*. 1998;4:331-334.

forms a complex on the platelet membrane with Va and calcium and cleaves prothrombin to thrombin; this complex is termed the prothrombinase complex.

As is apparent from the above description, platelets play a critical role in thrombus formation (see Chapter 2, *Role of the Platelet*). Platelets become adherent to collagen exposed at the site of injury and platelets are also trapped in the developing thrombus. Platelets in both of these locations become activated and release membrane vesicles known as microparticles, which are highly thrombogenic.[7]

The soluble thrombin generated by platelets is a major contributor to clot formation and propagation.

Regulation of Thrombin Generation

Thrombin generation is limited by thrombomodulin (TM) (Figure 1.2).[8] TM binds thrombin, inhibiting its protease activity. The TM-thrombin complex then activates protein C (APC). APC inactivates VIIIa, and along with factor V and free protein S, inactivates Va. Protein S, a 64 kd glycoprotein, is present in free (40%) and bound (60%) forms; the binding protein (BP) of protein S is the fourth component of complement (C4B)-BP. It has recently been suggested that β2-glycoprotein-1, a phospholipid-binding protein, functions to inhibit binding of protein S by C4B-BP.[9] This would enhance the anticoagulant effect of protein S. Free protein S inhibits the tenase and prothrombinase complex by covering phospholipids on the cell membrane. In addition, the inactivation of VIIIa and Va by APC helps to limit thrombin generation.[10-12]

Fibrin Generation

Thrombin converts fibrinogen to fibrin and activates factor XIII (XIIIa) (Figure 1.3).[13] Fibrinogen is a 340 kd glycoprotein composed of a dimer of three polypeptide chains. Thrombin cleaves the amino-termini of the α- and β-chains, releasing fibrinopeptides A and B, converting fibrinogen to fibrin monomer. The monomers spontaneously aggregate, forming protofibrils. XIIIa cross-links the fibrils to solidify the clot.

Fibrinolysis

Circulating plasminogen binds to the fibrin clot and is converted to plasmin by tissue plasminogen activator (tPA) (Figure 1.4),[14] which is released from the endothelium and binds to fibrin. Fibrinolysis is also activated by the contact activation system.[15] As noted previously, PK converts prourokinase to urokinase, which in turn activates plasminogen to plasmin. Plasmin dissolves fibrin, resulting in clot

FIGURE 1.2 — REGULATION OF THROMBIN ACTIVITY

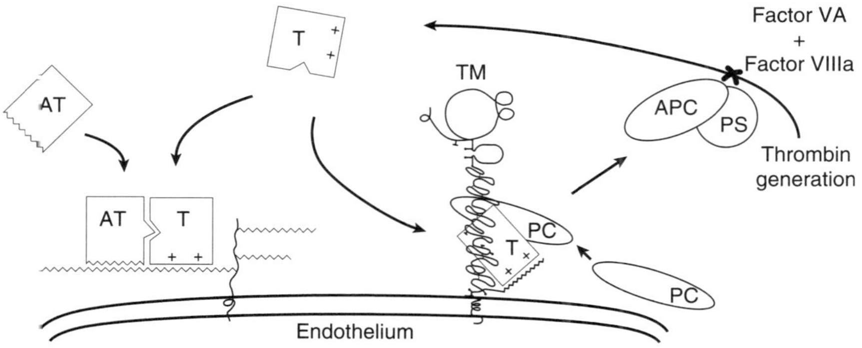

To the left is heparan sulfate proteoglycan, to which thrombin (T) and antithrombin (AT) bind. To the right is thrombomodulin (TM) which acts as a receptor for T. The TM+T complex activates protein C (PC) to activated protein C (APC). APC with protein S (PS) as a cofactor inactivates factor Va and VIIIa, which in turn downregulates T generation.

Bourin MC, Lindahl U. *Biochem J.* 1993;289(pt 2):313-330, and Dahlback B, Stenflo J. The protein C anticoagulant system. In: Stamatoyannopoulos G Nienhuis AW, Majerus PW, Varmus H, eds. *Molecular Basis of Blood Diseases.* 2nd ed. Philadelphia, Pa: WB Saunders; 1994:599-627.

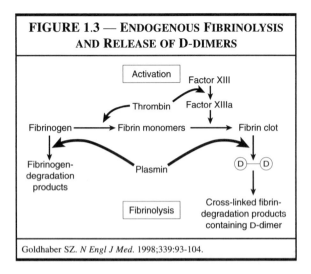

FIGURE 1.3 — ENDOGENOUS FIBRINOLYSIS AND RELEASE OF D-DIMERS

Activation

Factor XIII

Thrombin → Factor XIIIa

Fibrinogen → Fibrin monomers → Fibrin clot

Fibrinogen-degradation products ← Plasmin

(D)—(D)

Fibrinolysis

Cross-linked fibrin-degradation products containing D-dimer

Goldhaber SZ. *N Engl J Med.* 1998;339:93-104.

lysis. Activated platelets and endothelial cells release plasminogen activator inhibitor-1, and XIIIa cross-links α2-antiplasmin to the fibrin clot. These two inhibitors act to control fibrinolysis. In addition, thrombin in the presence of TM activates a potent inhibitor of fibrinolysis designated thrombin activatable fibrinolysis inhibitor (TAFI).[16,17]

Vascular Factors in Thrombus Formation

The hemostatic reactions described above occur in the setting of pulsatile blood flow, a vascular system lined by endothelium, and a milieu consisting of a variety of cells, cell fragments, and proteins.[18] Blood flow produces different shear stresses within the vasculature; on the arterial side of the circulation, platelets are driven against the vessel wall and are the principal component of thrombi (white thrombus), whereas on the venous side, thrombi consist mainly of fibrin and red cells, with platelets passively deposited. Under high shear stresses, adherence of platelets to the subendothelium is dependent on the binding of von Willebrand's factor (vWf) to platelet receptors. von Willebrand's factor is also critical for platelet aggregation. Another role of vWf is as a carrier protein for factor VIII.

FIGURE 1.4 — COMPONENTS OF THE FIBRINOLYTIC SYSTEM

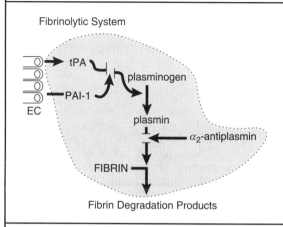

Tissue-type plasminogen activator (tPA) is released from endothelial cells (EC), where it binds to the fibrin clot (shaded area). Plasminogen activator inhibitor-1 (PAI-1) inhibits the action of tPA. Following its generation from plasminogen, plasmin lyses fibrin, but is inhibited by α_2-antiplasmin.

LS Lessin. *Medical Knowledge Self-Assessment Program, Hematology.* Philadelphia, Pa: American College of Physicians. 1994:203.

Factor VIII is resistant to inactivation by APC while it remains associated with the vWf.

The endothelium plays multiple roles in hemostasis, contributing factors that inhibit platelet aggregation, inactivate thrombin, and mediate clot lysis.[19] For example, endothelial cells are a rich source of prostacyclin and nitric oxide, which inhibit platelet aggregation and are potent vasodilators. Dermatan sulfate, a vessel-wall proteoglycan, binds heparin cofactor II, and the complex inactivates clot-bound thrombin. The endothelium also releases tPA.[20]

Summary

All coagulation reactions take place on a negatively charged surface, the membrane of activated platelets. Thus platelets play a critical role in thrombin generation (see Chapter 2, *Role of the Platelet*).[21] Procoagulant complexes bind to specific platelet phospholipids, vWf adheres to membrane glycoproteins (GP) Ib and IIb/IIIa, and GPIb may act as a fibrin receptor. Leukocytes adhere to activated platelets and secrete cytokines and expose tissue factor, which further amplifies hemostasis. Under pathologic conditions, the shedding of negatively charged membrane microparticles from erythrocytes and macrophages also enhances coagulation reactions. Modulating these processes are a vast number of physiologic antithrombotic mechanisms, which include circulating anticoagulants, such as proteins C and S, antithrombin, β_2-glycoprotein-1 and annexins; endothelium-derived factors, such as TFPI, TM, prostacyclin, and nitric oxide; and fibrinolytic agents, including tPA, urokinase, and plasminogen. As Virchow noted more than 100 years ago, the vessel wall, the character of blood flow, and the composition of the blood all play a role in thrombus formation.[22]

REFERENCES

1. Mann KG, Gaffney D, Bovill EG. Molecular biology, biochemistry, and lifespan of plasma coagulation factors. In: Beutler E, Lichtmen MA, Coller VS, eds. *Williams Hematology*. 5th ed. New York, NY: McGraw-Hill, Inc; 1994:1206.

2. Broze GJ Jr. The tissue factor pathway of coagulation. In: Loscalzo J, Schafer AI, eds. *Thrombosis and Hemorrhage*. 2nd ed. Baltimore, Md: Williams and Wilkins; 1998:77-104.

3. Roberts HR, Monroe DM, Oliver JA, Chang JY, Hoffman M. Newer concepts of blood coagulation. *Haemophilia*. 1998;4:331-334.

4. Colman RW. Biologic activities of the contact factors in vivo. *Thromb Haemost*. 1999;82:1568-1577.

5. Walsh PN. Platelets and factor XI bypass the contact system of blood coagulation. *Thromb Haemost*. 1999;82:234-242.

6. Martincic D, Kravtsov V, Gailani D. Factor XI messenger RNA in human platelets. *Blood*. 1999;94:3397-3404.

7. Ilveskero S, Siljander P, Lassila R. Procoagulant activity on platelets adhered to collagen or plasma clot. *Arterioscler Thromb Vasc Biol*. 2001;21:628-635.

8. Simmonds RE, Lane DA. Regulation of coagulation. In: Loscalzo J, Schafer AI, eds. *Thrombosis and Hemorrhage*. 2nd ed. Baltimore, Md: Williams and Wilkins; 1998:46.

9. Merrill JT, Zhang HW, Shen C, et al. Enhancement of protein S anticoagulant function by β_2-glycoprotein 1, a major target antigen of antiphospholipid antibodies. *Thromb Haemost*. 1999;81:748-757.

10. Smirnov MD, Safa O, Esmon NL, Esmon CT. Inhibition of activated protein C anticoagulant activity by prothrombin. *Blood*. 1999; 94:3839-3846.

11. Han X, Fiehler R, Broze GJ. Characterization of protein Z-dependent protease inhibitor. *Blood*. 2000;96:3049-3055.

12. Rezaie AR. Prothrombin protects factor Xa in the prothrombinase complex from inhibition by the heparin-antithrombin complex. *Blood*. 2001;97:2308-2313.

13. Goldhaber SZ. Pulmonary embolism. *N Engl J Med*. 1998;339:93-104.

14. Hemostasis and thrombosis. In: Lessin LS, ed. *Medical Knowledge Self-Assessment Program, Hematology*. Philadelphia, Pa: American College of Physicians; 1994:203.

15. Gaffney PJ, Edgell TA, Whitton CM. The haemostatic balance—Astrup revisited. *Haemostasis*. 1999;29:58-71.

16. Bajzar L, Manuel R, Nesheim ME. Purification and characterization of TAFI, a thrombin-activable fibrinolysis inhibitor. *J Biol Chem*. 1995;270:14477-14484.

17. Bouma BN, Meijers JCM. Fibrinolysis and the contact system: a role for factor XI in the down-regulation of fibrinolysis. *Thromb Haemost*. 1999;82:243-250.

18. Fuster V, Fayad ZA, Badimon JJ. Acute coronary syndromes: biology. *Lancet*. 1999;353(suppl 2):S5-S9.

19. Bombeli T, Mueller M, Haeberli A. Anticoagulant properties of the vascular endothelium. *Thromb Haemost*. 1997;77:408-423.

20. Rosenberg RD, Aird WC. Vascular-bed—specific hemostasis and hypercoagulable states. *N Engl J Med*. 1999;340:1333-1364.

21. Beguin S, Keularts I. On the coagulation of platelet-rich plasma. *Haemostasis*. 1999;29:50-57.

22. Virchow RLK. *Thrombosis and Emboli* (1846-1856). Matzdorff AC, Bell WR, trans. Canton, Mass: Science History Publications; 1998:234.

2   Role of the Platelet

Platelets are recognized for their essential role in vascular hemostasis, but in addition they contribute directly to pathologic thrombosis, particularly events occurring within the arterial circulatory system in regions of high shear stress and at sites of atheromatous plaque disruption.

Platelet Physiology

Under normal physiologic conditions, platelets circulate freely within the cardiovascular system, avoiding meaningful interactions with other cells and the vessel wall. The circumstances are distinctly different following vascular injury, which elicits a rapid change in platelet behavior that can be either lifesaving or life-threatening, depending on the site of involvement, degree of response, and the functional capability of regulatory pathways.

The role of platelets in arterial thrombosis is best appreciated in the context of five important physiologic steps (Figure 2.1):

- Platelet adhesion
- Platelet activation
- Platelet secretion
- Platelet aggregation
- Platelet support of coagulation.

■ Platelet Adhesion

For platelets to contribute meaningfully to the thrombotic process, they must first "stick" or adhere to sites of vessel-wall damage. This important initiating step is mediated by specific surface receptors that are recognized by adhesive proteins (ligands) residing on or near to the vascular endothelial surface.[1] In the case of platelet adhesion, the critical components are:

- von Willebrand factor (vWf)
- Glycoprotein (GP) Ib-IX-V complex.

FIGURE 2.1 — CHAIN OF EVENTS IN ARTERIAL THROMBOSIS

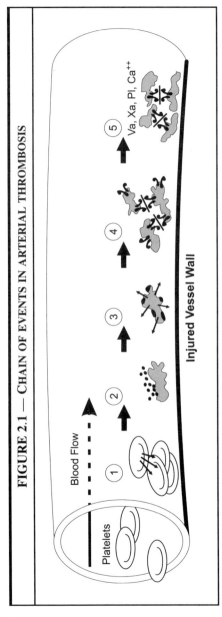

Abbreviations: Ca^{++}, calcium; Pl, phospholipid.

Chain of events in arterial thrombosis: 1) platelets *adhere* to sites of vessel wall injury (via von Willebrand factor bound to the GPIb/IX/V receptor complex); 2) *activation* elicits a conformational change that stimulates intracellular events and provokes microparticle release; 3) *secretion* of intracellular contents from α-granules, dense bodies, and lysosomes prepares the platelet for cellular events to follow; 4) *aggregation* is achieved through the fibrinogen-mediated binding of adjacent platelets via GPIIb/IIIa receptors, and; 5) the platelet aggregates provide a surface for *coagulation protease assembly*, thrombin generation, and fibrin formation.

Under high shear stress conditions, vWf can also bind the platelet GPIIb/IIIa receptor.

■ Platelet Activation

Following adhesion, platelets become *activated* in response to a wide variety of biochemical and mechanical stimuli.[2] Of physiologic relevance, many of the agonists are themselves a product of platelets that are released, initiating several strong and repetitive "positive feedback" or "bioamplification" reactions.

Platelet agonists bind surface GPs and stimulate signal transduction across the membrane via specific messenger proteins that, in turn, trigger either one or two intracellular pathways—the phosphoinositide pathway (leading to calcium mobilization and surface expression of GPIIb/IIIa receptors) and the phospholipase A_2—arachidonate pathway (stimulating the production of thromboxane A_2 generation).

Platelet activation, in addition to its biochemical effects, results in physical changes that facilitate platelet–vessel-wall binding, platelet aggregation, and platelet-leukocyte interactions. The formation of microparticles expands the prothrombotic surface area substantially.

■ Platelet Secretion

Platelet activation stimulates intracellular calcium mobilization, surface receptor expression (ligand-receptive conformational change), and the secretion of contents from three distinct storage granules—lysosomes, α-granules, and dense bodies.[3]

Lysosomes contain a variety of acid hydrolases that digest endocytotic materials but do not play a pivotal role in arterial thrombosis. In contrast, dense bodies house adenosine diphosphate, serotonin, and calcium, each an important component of the thrombotic process. Similarly, platelet α-granules are an important storage site for platelet-specific proteins (platelet-derived growth factors), coagulation factors (factor V, fibrinogen), and GPs (thrombospondin, GPIIb/IIIa).

■ Platelet Aggregation

The adhered and activated platelets in essence are primed for aggregation and, in so doing, provide a "plug" for localized vascular injury and a template for further thrombus growth. Platelet aggregation is mediated predominantly by fibrinogen (a dimeric GP found in abundance within plasma and α-granules) that binds surface GPIIb/IIIa receptors with high affinity (>40,000 molecules per cell), bridging adjacent platelets.

Sequences of the fibrinogen molecule that bind the platelet GPIIb/IIIa receptor have been identified on its Aα (RGDF) and δ (RGDS) chains. Other proteins that contribute to platelet aggregation, particularly under high shear stress conditions include vWf, fibronectin, and vitronectin.

Because platelet aggregation is regulated by the GPIIb/IIIa receptor, it has become a favored target for pharmacologic therapies used in the management of acute coronary syndromes.[4-6]

- **Platelet Support of Coagulation**

Aggregated platelets deposited at a site of vessel-wall injury form a physiologically ideal template for thrombus growth and stabilization. The second phase of arterial thrombosis (in contrast to the first phase culminating with platelet aggregation) is mediated by coagulation proteases that assemble on the platelet surface and facilitate thrombin generation and fibrin formation. Dysfunctional endothelial cells and possibly monocytes can also support prothrombinase complex assembly.

Summary

The platelet is a structurally and functionally complex component of protective hemostasis and vascular thrombosis occurring at localized sites of injury. Platelet adherence, activation, secretion, and aggregation collectively define the primary phase of thrombosis, while assembly and initiation of the coagulation cascade and, ultimately, fibrin formation represent the second or growth phase. The defining steps for thrombosis are governed by surface receptors and adhesive proteins that provide potential targets for pharmacologic intervention designed to either prevent or, at the very least, attenuate the thrombotic response to vessel-wall injury.

REFERENCES

1. Phillips DR, Agin PP. Platelet plasma membrane glycoproteins. Evidence for the presence of nonequivalent disulfide bonds using nonreduced-reduced two-dimensional gel electrophoresis. *J Biol Chem.* 1977;252:2121-2126.

2. Berridge MJ. Inositol triphosphate and diacylglycerol: two interacting second messengers. *Annu Rev Biochem.* 1987;56:159-193.

3. Stenberg PE, Shuman MA, Levine SP, Bainton DF. Redistribution of alpha-granules and their contents in thrombin-stimulated platelets. *J Cell Biol.* 1984;98:748-760.

4. Farrell DH, Thiagarajan P, Chung DW, Davie EW. Role of fibrinogen alpha and gamma chain sites in platelet aggregation. *Proc Natl Acad Sci USA.* 1992;89:10729-10732.

5. Byzova TV, Plow EF. Networking in the hemostatic system. *J Biol Chem.* 1997;272:27183-27188.

6. Lefkovits J, Plow EF, Topol EJ. Platelet glycoprotein IIb/IIIa receptors in cardiovascular medicine. *N Engl J Med.* 1995;332:1553-1559.

3

Heparins, Direct Thrombin Inhibitors, and Warfarin

Heparin

Heparin is a highly charged polyanion consisting of chains of 18 to 50 saccharide units.[1] Since each saccharide has a molecular weight of about 300 d, the overall molecular weight of the compound ranges from 5000 to 30,000 d, with a mean of 15,000 d. About one third of the chains have a specific pentasaccharide sequence that binds antithrombin; the larger chains also bind thrombin, dramatically enhancing the ability of antithrombin to inactivate thrombin.

Heparin also binds to a variety of cells and plasma proteins. The former include macrophages and platelets, and the latter are fibrinogen, vitronectin, fibronectin, and von Willebrand factor among others. Heparin also has a strong affinity for platelet factor 4 exposed on the surface of activated platelets. As a consequence of these various interactions, there is dose-dependent absorption from subcutaneous injection sites and highly variable plasma levels, depending on the concentration of heparin-binding proteins. Furthermore, there is a dose-dependent half-life; as little as 56 minutes after a dose of 100 U/kg and as long as 156 min after 400 U/kg. Because of these pharmacologic characteristics, it is difficult to predict the dose of heparin that may be safe and effective in a given patient. Therefore, the dose must be titrated by trial and error, using the activated partial thromboplastin time (aPTT) as a guide (see Chapter 9, *Monitoring of Anticoagulants*).

By virtue of its ability to potentiate the anticoagulant effects of antithrombin, heparin promotes the inactivation of thrombin and activated clotting factors XI, X, IX, and the tissue factor—factor VIIa complex. This results in prolongation of the aPTT, prothrombin time (PT), and thrombin time. The most sensitive to the effects of heparin are the thrombin time and aPTT; the PT is affected by heparin concentrations greater than 0.5 U/mL. Although heparin has a strong inhibitory effect on thrombin in plasma, the heparin-antithrombin complex is unable to inhibit thrombin bound to fibrin. This becomes important when lytic treatment is given; as thrombi lyse, fibrin-bound thrombin is able to continue converting fibrinogen to fibrin despite the presence of heparin, leading to rethrombosis.

Heparin has a number of other effects in addition to its binding of antithrombin. It impairs bone formation and enhances bone resorption; in susceptible persons, prolonged administration of the drug may lead to osteoporosis and fractures. Its binding to platelet factor 4 may stimulate antibody formation, resulting in heparin-induced thrombocytopenia (HIT). In concentrations greater than 0.5 U/mL, it alters platelet function and increases vascular permeability. Heparin also has inhibitory activity toward aldosterone, manifest by a mildly increased serum potassium.

Low Molecular Weight Heparin

Low molecular weight heparin (LMWH) is prepared by the depolymerization of porcine heparin. A variety of proprietary processes are used, giving distinctive products whose molecular weights range from 4000 to 6500 d, and number of saccharide units, from 13 to 22.[2] As with unfractionated heparin (UFH), about one third of the LMWH chains have the pentasaccharide binding site for antithrombin, but unlike heparin, only chains having 18 or more saccharide units bind thrombin. Thus the LMWH-antithrombin complex has weak antithrombin activity but retains the ability to inactivate factor Xa. The ratio of anti-Xa activity to anti-IIa (antithrombin) activity varies from 2:1 to 4:1. Because of its weak effect on thrombin, LMWH only prolongs the aPTT when present in very high plasma concentrations. This raises the question of why LMWH is an effective anticoagulant. LMWH releases tissue factor pathway inhibitor (TFPI) from endothelium; TFPI binds factor Xa and inhibits the tissue factor—factor VIIa complex. In addition, complexes of LMWH and antithrombin are able to inactivate factor Xa bound to platelets. However, similar to heparin, LMWH is not able to inhibit thrombin bound to fibrin.[3]

When LMWH is given in either fixed or weight-adjusted doses by the subcutaneous route, greater than 90% of the dose is absorbed. In contrast to heparin, LMWH has minimal binding to cells or plasma proteins, resulting in persistence of free drug in the circulation and a longer half-life of activity. While the half-life of UFH averages about 90 minutes, the half-lives of three LMWHs range from 108 to 252 minutes. Studies have also demonstrated that the effect of LMWH on factor Xa activity is linearly related to the dose administered. These pharmacologic characteristics mean that plasma levels are predictable and monitoring is unnecessary in most patients.[4] Anti-Xa activity can be detected in the plasma of most patients receiving LMWH, but the levels may not predict clinical efficacy. On the other hand, plasma anti-Xa concentrations greater than 1.0 U/mL may be associated with bleeding. Therefore, it is prudent to monitor anti-Xa levels in patients in whom high levels of drug may be anticipated. These would include children weighing less than 50 kg or persons of more than 120 kg receiving weight-adjusted doses. Pregnant women and patients with renal failure should also be monitored; the former because their doses may be changing as the pregnancy progresses and they gain weight, and the latter because LMWH is largely excreted by the kidneys.

Thrombocytopenia is infrequently associated with LMWH, but antibodies directed against complexes of LMWH and platelet factor 4 can be detected in some patients. On rare occasion, the full-blown syndrome of heparin-induced thrombocytopenia occurs. Equally rare is necrosis at the site of skin injections with LMWH, which may be a form of local HIT. LMWH inhibits bone formation but does not enhance bone resorption in laboratory studies. Clinically, osteoporosis appears to be less frequent with LMWH than with UFH, based on investigation of bone density in pregnant women receiving these anticoagulants.

Bleeding is the major adverse effect of heparin and LMWH. It most commonly appears at the sites of trauma; for example, the inguinal area in patients having femoral vessel catheterization. The most feared complication is epidural bleeding and spinal hematoma following insertion or removal of an epidural catheter inserted to provide perioperative anesthesia.[5] The frequency of bleeding appears to be less with LMWH than with UFH, based on a meta-analysis of thirteen studies comparing the two in the treatment of deep vein thrombosis.[7] The following factors increase the risk of bleeding:

- Low body weight
- Age over 70 years
- Recent surgery or trauma
- Concomitant use of drugs that affect hemostasis such as fibrinolytic agents or inhibitors of platelet function.

The latter include not only aspirin but also nonsteroidal antiinflammatory agents. The antidote for bleeding due to UFH is protamine; this agent may also be used for bleeding associated with LMWH, but is less effective.

A number of LMWHs are currently available or under development. The manufacturing process for each drug differs from that for the others, and each has pharmacologic properties that are modestly different. Whether these differences affect the safety and efficacy of an individual agent is unknown. However, based on the properties of their LMWH, manufacturers have recommended varying dosage regimens (Tables 3.1 and 3.2). For example, enoxaparin is dosed in milligrams and given either once or twice daily, whereas dalteparin and tinzaparin are dosed in units and usually given once daily. While some LMWHs are given in fixed doses for prophylaxis, tinzaparin is almost always dosed based on body weight. Danaparoid is given in a fixed dose of 750 U twice daily for prophylaxis after hip-replacement surgery. Because of their high degree of bioavailability, all LMWHs are given subcutaneously. The LMWHs and heparinoids currently (October 2001) approved by the Food and Drug Administration (FDA) for the prophylaxis of venous thromboembolism are shown in Table 3.1.

All LMWHs are given in higher doses for treatment indications such as the therapy of venous thrombosis or the management of unstable angina. Those currently approved by the FDA are shown in Table 3.2. In addition, many LMWHs have been used for a variety of other clinical conditions including stroke (both thromboprophylaxis and treatment), neurosurgery (prevention of postoperative thromboembolism), and thromboprophylaxis after trauma, includ-

TABLE 3.1 — CURRENTLY AVAILABLE LMWHS AND HEPARINOIDS FOR THROMBOPROPHYLAXIS

Drug (Trade)	Dose	Indication
Enoxaparin (Lovenox)	30 mg q 12 h; 40 mg daily	Medical inpatients; Hip/knee/abdominal surgery
Dalteparin (Fragmin)	2500 U q 12 h; 5000 U daily	Hip/abdominal surgery
Danaparoid (Orgaran)	750 U q 12 h	Hip surgery
Abbreviations: LMWH, low molecular weight heparin.		

ing spinal cord injury and hip fracture.[6] They have also been used for the prevention of thrombi in vascular grafts and fistulae. Although these uses are not FDA-approved as yet, LMWH is gradually supplanting UFH because of its:

- Convenience (once or twice daily subcutaneous injections)
- Lack of need for routine monitoring
- Overall high degree of safety.[7,8]

Pentasaccharide

The five saccharide chain that binds and activates antithrombin has recently been synthesized and studied as a thromboprophylactic agent.[9-12] It has a number of potential advantages over LMWH: no interaction with platelets and therefore no risk of HIT; not made from any animal products; and the possibility of greater efficacy and safety. In studies of patients with hip fracture and hip or knee replacement surgery, pentasaccharide was more effective than enoxaparin when used in a dose of 2.5 mg subcutaneously daily, and with a similar rate of bleeding. A disadvantage may be higher cost because of the complex chemical synthesis required and a very long plasma half-life. Further trials examining this promising new agent are underway.

TABLE 3.2 — CURRENT FDA-APPROVED LMWHS FOR TREATMENT*

Drug (Trade)	Dose	Indication
Dalteparin (Fragmin)	120 IU/kg q12h	Treatment of unstable angina and non–ST-segment elevation myocardial infarction for the prevention of ischemic complications in patients on concurrent aspirin therapy.
Enoxaparin (Lovenox)	1 mg/kg q12h; 1.5 mg/kg daily	Prevention of ischemic complications of unstable angina and non–ST-segment elevation myocardial infarction when concurrently administered with aspirin; inpatient treatment of acute DVT with and without PE when administered in conjunction with warfarin; outpatient treatment with acute DVT without PE when administered in conjunction with warfarin.
Tinzaparin (Innohep)	175 IU/kg daily	Inpatient treatment of acute DVT with and without PE when administered in conjunction with warfarin.

* All given subcutaneously.

Abbreviations: DVT, deep venous thrombosis; FDA, Food and Drug Administration; LMWH, low molecular weight heparin; PE, pulmonary embolism.

Hirudin

Hirudin is a product of the medicinal leech, *Hirudo medicinalis*, but is currently prepared by recombinant DNA technology. Three forms have been examined clinically:
- Recombinant hirudin (lepirudin, desirudin)
- Hirugen
- Bivalirudin.

Hirudin binds to both the catalytic site and the fibrinogen-binding exosite of thrombin, hirugen binds only to the exosite, and bivalirudin is a synthetic peptide (20 amino acids) that binds to both the catalytic site and the exosite.[13] Hirudin has been further modified by conjugation with polyethylene glycol (PEG-hirudin), which has a longer half-life than hirudin. The half-life of hirudin is 50 to 65 minutes, with a half-life of its effect on the aPTT of 2 hours.[14] Bivalirudin has a half-life of effect on the aPTT of about 40 minutes.[15] The pharmacologic advantages and disadvantages of the hirudins as compared with the heparins are shown in Table 3.3.

Hirudins form a tight complex with thrombin, inhibiting thrombin conversion of fibrinogen to fibrin as well as thrombin-induced platelet aggregation.[16] These actions are independent of the presence of antithrombin, and also affect thrombin bound to fibrin. On the downside, the ability of thrombin to complex with thrombomodulin, activating protein C, is also inhibited. The hirudins do not bind to platelet factor 4 and do not elicit antibodies that induce platelet and endothelial cell activation; thus they may be safely administered to patients that have developed HIT. Hirudins do have weak immunogenicity, so that diminished (or rarely increased) responsiveness after repeated dosing is possible. The aPTT is prolonged and is used to monitor the effect of the hirudins. The prothrombin time is modestly prolonged, which may interfere with the monitoring of concomitant warfarin therapy. Hirudin rapidly increases to toxic levels in patients with renal failure; the doses must be halved or further reduced in such patients. While protamine effectively reverses the anticoagulant effect of UFH, and is also partially effective in neutralizing LMWH, there is no antidote for hirudins except plasma exchange. Two

TABLE 3.3 — PROPERTIES OF HEPARINS AND HIRUDINS		
Property	**Heparins**	**Hirudins**
Thrombin inhibition	Require AT	Directly inhibit
Clot-bound thrombin	Not inhibited	Inhibited
Thrombocytopenia	Yes	No
Immunogenicity	Absent	Weak
Effect on aPTT	Yes (weak with LMWH)	Yes
Effect on PT	Weak	Moderate
Metabolism	Liver, kidney	Kidney
Antidote	Protamine*	None

Abbreviations: aPTT, activated partial thromboplastin time; AT, antithrombin; LMWH, low molecular weight heparin; PT, prothrombin time.

* 60% reversal of LMWH.

preparations, a recombinant hirudin (lepirudin [Refludan]) and hirulog (bivalirudin [Angiomax]), have been licensed in the United States. Lepirudin is used for the management of HIT, and bivalirudin is indicated for patients with unstable angina undergoing percutaneous coronary intervention (PCI). In randomized clinical trials of patients undergoing PCI, the frequency of death, myocardial infarction, and need for revascularization procedures was 6.2% in those treated with bivalirudin and 7.9% for those receiving heparin; the frequency of major hemorrhage was less with bivalirudin (3.5% vs 9.3%). The drug is always administered with aspirin; its safety in conjunction with platelet glycoprotein IIb/IIIa inhibitors is under investigation.

Argatroban is a small molecule thrombin inhibitor with properties similar to the hirudins (Table 3.3). However, an important difference is that it is metabolized by the liver rather than the kidney and therefore may be given without dose adjustment to patients with renal failure. The starting dose is 2 µg/kg/min; the aPTT is checked at 4 hours and the dose adjusted until the target aPTT of 1.5 to 3.0 times the control is attained. The dose is decreased by 0.5 µg/kg/min if there is hepatic impairment. The drug is approved for the management of HIT. Like the hirudins, argatroban can modestly prolong the prothrombin time, necessitating dose adjustments when warfarin is given concomitantly (see Chapter 18, *Complications of Antithrombotic Therapy*).

Warfarin (Coumadin)

Coumarins inhibit the enzymatic reduction of vitamin K epoxide. Vitamin K (in the reduced state) is the coenzyme of a carboxylase responsible for the carboxylation of glutamic acid residues on factors II, VII, IX, and X and proteins C, S, and Z. The acarboxylated forms of these clotting proteins can be detected in the circulation of warfarin-treated patients but are inert with respect to coagulant activity.

Several coumarins have been developed for clinical use; acenocoumarol is available in Europe but not used in the United States, where warfarin is the most commonly used oral anticoagulant. Warfarin is rapidly absorbed from the gastrointestinal tract and has a half-life of 36 to 42 hours. After a dose of warfarin, the synthesis of carboxylated factors ceases, but the effects on coagulation will depend on the disappearance of carboxylated factors formed prior to warfarin exposure. The disappearance of these factors is a function of their half-life (factor VII and protein C: 6 to 7 hours; factors IX and X: 24 hours; prothrombin: 90 hours). Thus, after a dose of warfarin, factor VII and protein C will be 20% of normal at 48 hours, but prothrombin will not be reduced to this extent for 1 to 2 weeks. Since effective anticoagulation requires a decrease in clotting factors to 20% of normal, warfarin is considered a slow-acting anticoagulant.[17]

The effect of warfarin is monitored with the prothrombin time, which is sensitive to factors II, V, VII, and X. Although factor IX is not measured, it is usually reduced in parallel with factor X and therefore does not have to be separately quantitated. Clinical and laboratory studies suggest that prolongation of the prothrombin time to 1.5 to 2 times normal prevents the growth of a thrombus. The international normalized ratio (INR) refers to the ratio of patient-to-control prothrombin time raised to a power — the international sensitivity index (ISI). For example, if the prothrombin time is 1.5 times longer than the control prothrombin time and the ISI (of the prothrombin time reagent) is 2, the INR is 2.25 (1.5 raised to the power of 2). Values of 2 to 3 are considered therapeutic. Therefore, the dose of warfarin is titrated to give an INR in this range.

Warfarin is subject to extensive binding by plasma proteins and is metabolized by the P450 detoxification system of the liver. Persons with genetic polymorphisms of the CYP 2C9 enzyme may have impaired metabolism of warfarin and may require doses of the drug that are substantially less than those in persons with the wild type enzyme.[18] These polymorphisms occur in about one in ten white persons.[19] Drugs that alter protein binding or affect the liver may potentiate or inhibit the activity of warfarin (Table 3.4).[20] Acetaminophen has been shown to produce a dose-dependent increase in the INR of warfarin-treated patients, beginning with a dose as low as seven to thirteen 325-mg tablets per week.[21] Even herbal remedies such as ginkgo and ginseng, as well as numerous others, may alter warfarin metabolism.[22] Other factors found to affect warfarin were the dietary content of vitamin K, the ability to absorb vitamin K (altered by diarrheal disease), and advanced malignancy.

An important adverse reaction to warfarin therapy is tissue necrosis due to severely decreased levels of protein C or S. This complication occurs in patients with genetic mutations in proteins C and S, or in persons who lack these proteins because of vitamin K deficiency, often clinically unsuspected. When such individuals are exposed to warfarin, the sudden decline in proteins C and S leads to thrombus formation in venules with extensive skin and subcutaneous fat necrosis. Even more profound thrombosis, producing limb gangrene, occurs when warfarin is given to patients with HIT. The mechanism appears to be similar—an underlying deficiency in protein C that is exacerbated by the administration of warfarin.[23]

Other adverse effects attributed to warfarin are fetal embryopathy, especially with exposure to the drug from the sixth to twelfth weeks of gestation; and "purple toes," re-

TABLE 3.4 — LEVEL-1 EVIDENCE OF DRUG INTERACTIONS WITH WARFARIN

Interaction	Antibiotics	Cardiac	Anti-inflammatory	CNS	GI
Potentiate	Cotrimoxazole Erythromycin Fluconazole Isoniazid Metronidazole	Amiodarone Clofibrate Propafenone Propranolol Sulfinpyrazone	Phenylbutazone Piroxicam	Alcohol (with liver disease)	Cimetidine Omeprazole
Inhibit	Griseofulvin Nafcillin Rifampin	Cholestyramine		Barbiturates Carbamazepine Chlordiazepoxide	Sucralfate
No effect	Enoxacin	Atenolol Bumetanide Felodipine Metoprolol	Diflunisal Ketorolac Naproxen	Alcohol Fluoxetine Nitrazepam	Antacids Famotidine

Abbreviations: CNS, central nervous system; GI, gastrointestinal.

Wells PS, et al. *Ann Intern Med.* 1994;121:676-683.

3

lated to embolization of cholesterol-rich material from atheromatous aortic plaques.

A prolonged prothrombin time due to warfarin declines within 24 to 48 hours of drug discontinuation if the patient is eating. Vitamin K is the specific antidote: The dose is based on whether the patient is bleeding and the elevation of the INR, recognizing that the patient will be at risk for developing new thrombotic events if the INR is overcorrected and will be refractory to warfarin for several days if too large a dose is given. The dose of vitamin K is 1.0 mg to 2.5 mg orally for an INR of 5 to 10 in a nonbleeding patient; inability to eat, bleeding, or higher INR is managed with doses of 1 to 10 mg subcutaneously.[24] The intravenous route is reserved for patients with life-threatening hemorrhage, because vitamin K given by that route may cause anaphylaxis. In the event that bleeding is life-threatening, the clotting factors may be immediately replenished by giving plasma transfusions (15 mL/kg) or prothrombin complex concentrate (PCC) in doses of 50 U/kg.[25] Plasma will only partially correct the prothrombin time because of dilution effects but is less likely to promote thrombosis than is PCC. Because of the short half-life of factor VII, either plasma or PCC must be repeated every 4 to 6 hours to maintain correction of the prothrombin time.

Anticoagulants Currently Under Development

A large variety of compounds are currently under development; these include inhibitors of factors VIIa, IXa, Xa, and XIIIa and direct thrombin inhibitors. In addition, other anticoagulants are being reformulated so that they may be given by mouth. For example, an oral formulation of heparin is currently in clinical trials, and an oral thrombin inhibitor, ximelagatran, has shown promise in the prophylaxis of patients undergoing total knee replacement.[26] This agent has recently been compared with a traditional LMWH/warfarin regimen in the treatment of acute deep vein thrombosis.[27] Similar rates for regression of thrombus and major bleeding were seen with either treatment, suggesting that ximelagatran is an effective alternative to current antico-

agulant therapy. The eventual goal is to develop an anticoagulant that:

- Is easily administered
- Has a broad therapeutic index
- Does not require monitoring
- Can be used in the management of a wide variety of thrombotic disorders.

3

REFERENCES

1. Hirsh J. Heparin. *N Engl J Med*. 1991;324:1565-1574.

2. Hirsh J, Levine MN. Low molecular weight heparin. *Blood*. 1992;79:1-17.

3. Weitz JI. Low-molecular-weight heparins (published correction appears in *N Engl J Med*. 1997;337:1567.). *N Engl J Med*. 1997;337:688-698.

4. Laposata M, Green D, Van Cott EM, Barrowcliffe TW, Goodnight SH, Sosolik RE. College of American Pathologists Conference XXXI on Laboratory Monitoring of Anticoagulant Therapy: the clinical use and laboratory monitoring of low-molecular-weight heparin, danaparoid, hirudin and related compounds, and argatroban. *Arch Pathol Lab Med*. 1998;122:799-807.

5. Wysowski DX, Talarico L, Bacsanyi J, Botstein P. Spinal and epidural hematoma and low-molecular-weight heparin. *N Engl J Med*. 1998;338:1774-1775.

6. Green D, Hirsh J, Heit J, Prins M, Davidson B, Lensing AW. Low molecular weight heparin: a critical analysis of clinical trials. *Pharmacol Rev*. 1994;46:89-109.

7. Siguret V, Pautas E, Fevrier M, et al. Elderly patients treated with tinzaparin (Innohep) administered once daily (175 anti-Xa IU/kg): anti-Xa and anti-IIa activities over 10 days. *Thromb Haemost*. 2000;84:800-804.

8. Veiga F, Escriba A, Maluenda MP, et al. Low molecular weight heparin (enoxaparin) versus oral anticoagulant therapy (acenocoumarol) in the long-term treatment of deep venous thrombosis in the elderly: a randomized trial. *Thromb Haemost*. 2000;84:559-564.

9. Turpie AG, Gallus AS, Hoek JA. A synthetic pentasaccharide for the prevention of deep-vein thrombosis after total hip replacement. *N Engl J Med*. 2001;344:619-625.

10. Lassen MR. The Ephesus Study: comparison of the first synthetic factor Xa inhibitor with low molecular weight heparin in the prevention of venous thromboembolism after elective hip replacement surgery. *Blood*. 2000;96:490a.

11. Eriksson B. The Penthifra Study: comparison of the first synthetic factor Xa inhibitor with low molecular weight heparin in the prevention of venous thromboembolism after hip fracture surgery. *Blood*. 2000;96:490a.

12. Bauer K. The Pentamaks Study: comparison of the first synthetic factor Xa inhibitor with low molecular weight heparin in the prevention of venous thromboembolism after elective major knee surgery. *Blood*. 2000;96:490a.

13. Markwardt F. Hirudin and derivatives as anticoagulant agents. *Thromb Haemost*. 1991;66:141-152.

14. Verstraete M, Nurmohamed M, Kienast J, et al. Biologic effects of recombinant hirudin (CGP 39393) in human volunteers. European Hirudin in Thrombosis Group. *J Am Coll Cardiol*. 1993;22:1080-1088.

15. Fox I, Dawson A, Loynds P, et al. Anticoagulant activity of hirulog, a direct thrombin inhibitor in humans. *Thromb Haemost*. 1993;69:157-163.

16. Verstraete M. Direct thrombin inhibitors: appraisal of the antithrombotic/hemorrhagic balance. *Thromb Haemost*. 1997;78:357-363.

17. Hirsh J. Oral anticoagulant drugs. *N Engl J Med*. 1991;324:1865-1875.

18. Taube J, Halsall D, Baglin T. Influence of cytochrome P-450 CYP2C9 polymorphisms on warfarin sensitivity and risk of over-anticoagulation in patients on long-term treatment. *Blood*. 2000;96:1816-1819.

19. Xie HG, Kim RB, Wood AJ, Stein CM. Molecular basis of ethnic differences in drug disposition and response. *Annu Rev Pharmacol Toxicol*. 2001;41:815-850.

20. Wells PS, Holbrook AM, Crowther NR, Hirsh J. Interactions of warfarin with drugs and food. *Ann Intern Med*. 1994;121:676-683.

21. Hylek EM, Heiman H, Skates SJ, Sheehan MA, Singer DE. Acetaminophen and other risk factors for excessive warfarin anticoagulation. *JAMA*. 1998;279:657-662.

22. Fugh-Berman A. Herb-drug interactions. *Lancet*. 2000;355:134-138.

23. Warkentin TE, Elavathil LJ, Hayward CP, Johnston MA, Russett JI, Kelton JG. The pathogenesis of venous limb gangrene associated with heparin-induced thrombocytopenia. *Ann Intern Med.* 1997;127:804-812.

24. Weibert RT, Le DT, Kayser SR, Rapaport SI. Correction of excessive anticoagulation with low-dose oral vitamin K1. *Ann Intern Med.* 1997;125:959-962.

25. Makris M, Greaves M, Phillips WS, Kitchen S, Rosendaal FR, Preston EF. Emergency oral anticoagulant reversal: the relative efficacy of infusions of fresh frozen plasma and clotting factor concentrate on correction of the coagulopathy. *Thromb Haemost.* 1997;77:477-480.

26. Heit HA, Colwell CW, Francis CW, Ginsberg JS, Whipple J, Peters G. Comparison of the oral direct thrombin inhibitor H 376/95 with enoxaparin as prophylaxis against venous thromboembolism after total knee replacement: a phase II dose-finding study. *Blood.* 2000;96:491a.

27. Erikkson H, Wahlander K, Gustafsson D, Welin L, Frison L, Schulman S. Efficacy and tolerability of the novel, oral direct thrombin inhibitor, ximelagatran (pINN, formerly H 376/95), compared with standard therapy for the treatment of acute deep vein thrombosis. *Thromb Haemost.* 2001;(suppl). Abstract OC2348.

4   Fibrinolytic Agents

Recognizing the impact of acute thrombotic coronary arterial occlusion has led to a new paradigm: rapid, complete, and sustained patency of an occluded artery and physiologic myocardial perfusion. Fibrinolytic agents promote the conversion of plasminogen to plasmin, which then proteolytically degrades fibrin, the structural meshwork of an arterial thrombus.

Overview of the Fibrinolytic System

The exogenous fibrinolytic system is an important component of natural vascular thromboresistance, preventing thrombus mass beyond that required for hemostasis. Plasminogen is converted to plasmin, an enzyme that proteolytically degrades fibrin (Figures 4.1 and 4.2). Circulating plasmin inhibitors, particularly alpha$_2$-antiplasmin, rapidly inactivate free plasmin; however, when the rate of generation of plasmin exceeds the rate of inhibition, a systemic lytic state may ensue, with depletion of clotting factors, including fibrinogen, factor V, and factor VIII.[2] The natural plasminogen activators tissue plasminogen activator (tPA) and single-chain urokinase plasminogen activator (scu-PA) have fibrin-specific properties, suggesting that physiologic fibrinolysis is clot selective.[1]

Tissue Plasminogen Activator

Tissue plasminogen activator, produced by vascular endothelial cells and released in response to developing thrombus, is a naturally occurring 70,000 dalton glycoprotein (Figure 4.2). The native molecule is a single-chain polypeptide, but is converted to the fully active two-chain enzyme by plasmin-mediated cleavage (Figure 4.2 with an arrow). This unique structure, particularly the second kringle and the finger domain, confers high fibrin-specificity.[1] Plasminogen activator inhibitor can rapidly inactivate

FIGURE 4.1 — PATHWAYS OF THROMBOLYSIS

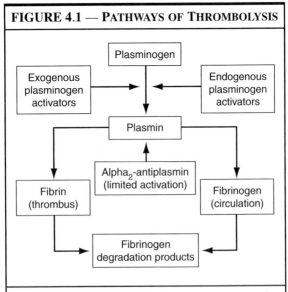

Endogenous or exogenous plasminogen activators convert plasminogen to the active serine protease plasmin, which degrades fibrin in thrombi and circulating fibrinogen. Plasmin in the circulation is rapidly inactivated by alpha$_2$-antiplasmin.

circulating tPA. In the absence of fibrin, tPA has weak enzymatic activity; however, when bound, tPA undergoes a conformational change that increases its plasmin-producing capacity by nearly 1000-fold. Thus plasmin is formed preferentially at the site of a developing thrombus (Figure 4.3).

Recombinant DNA technology was harnessed to produce alteplase, synthesized using the complementary DNA from natural human tPA. Alteplase is administered intravenously, starting with a bolus of 15 mg, followed by a rapid infusion of 50 mg over 30 minutes and a slower infusion of up to 35 mg over 60 minutes.[3,4] The rate of patency (Thrombolysis in Myocardial Infarction [TIMI] 2-3 flow) at 90 minutes is approximately 75% to 80%; full perfusion (TIMI-3 flow) occurs in approximately 55% of patients using a front-loaded regimen.[5] Table 4.1 summarizes the pharmacokinetic profile of alteplase. The plasma half-

FIGURE 4.2 — CHEMICAL STRUCTURE OF TISSUE PLASMINOGEN ACTIVATOR

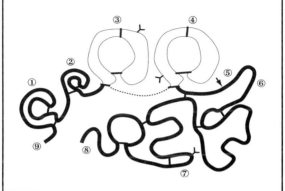

Domains and other molecular features: 1) finger domain, 2) growth factor domain, 3) kringle 1 domain, 4) kringle 2 domain, 5) peptide bond 275-276, 6) protease domain, 7) glycosylation sites, 8) carboxy terminus, 9) amino terminus.

Tissue plasminogen activator (tPA) is a serine protease containing 527 amino acids, with a finger and growth factor domain, 2 kringles, a protease domain, and numerous glycosylation sites and peptide bonds.

life is short, on the order of 4 to 8 minutes, and has a high degree of clot selectivity, leading to sparing of physiologic clotting mechanisms and a mild degree of fibrinogen depletion. Intracranial hemorrhage occurs in 0.5% to 1% of patients, and major (non-intracranial) bleeding in approximately 5%.[3] Clinical reocclusion occurs in approximately 10% of patients. Alteplase has been evaluated in randomized trials involving over 100,000 patients, with documented reductions in mortality and infarct size and improved left ventricular function. Antithrombotic therapy with intravenous (IV) unfractionated heparin should be initiated simultaneously with tPA, with a target activated partial thromboplastin time (aPTT) of 50 to 70 seconds.[3] Antiplatelet therapy with aspirin (or clopidogrel in cases of true aspirin allergy) should also be given prior to IV infusion of alteplase. Enhanced antiplatelet therapy with glycoprotein

FIGURE 4.3 — MECHANISM OF ACTION OF TISSUE PLASMINOGEN ACTIVATOR

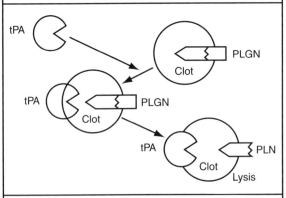

Tissue plasminogen activator (tPA) preferentially binds to fibrin, undergoing a conformational change that increases its ability to convert plasminogen (PLGN) to plasmin (PLN) up to 1000 fold.

(GP) IIb/IIIa receptor inhibitors has provided encouraging angiographic results with TIMI-3 flow rates of 80%.[6,7] The combined administration of tPA and enoxaparin is also an attractive alternative.

Streptokinase

Streptokinase (SK) is a bacterial protein secreted by group C beta-hemolytic streptococci. It was the first fibrinolytic agent developed for clinical use, with reports of clinical benefit in lysing clots within the pleural space more than 50 years ago, and the first description of use for myocardial infarction in 1954.[8] SK itself does not possess protease activity but must first bind to plasminogen, forming an activator complex which can then convert plasminogen to plasmin (Figure 4.4). The circulating half-life of SK is approximately 20 minutes. Because SK possesses only a modest degree of fibrin specificity, it activates both clot-bound plasminogen and circulating plasminogen. Free plasmin generated is rapidly inactivated by alpha$_2$-antiplasmin; however, once the capacity of this inhibitor is exhausted, re-

Feature	SK	APSAC	tPA	rPA	TNKase
Half-life (minutes)	25	100	6	15	20
Method of administration	1-hr IV	Bolus	1.5-hr IV	2 boluses	Bolus
Dose	1.5 mU/60 min	30 U	15 mg bolus, up to 85 mg/90 min	10+10 MU	0.55 mg/kg
Action	Indirect	Indirect	Direct	Direct	Direct
Fibrin specificity	NA	NA	NA	NA	NA
Antigenicity	+	+	++	+	+++
ICH rates	0.3%	0.7%	0.8%	0.8%	0.8%
Lives saved/1000	2.5	2.5	3.5	3-3.5	3.5
Cost ($US)	290	1700	2200	2200	2200
90-min TIMI 3 flow	~30%	~50%	~60%	~60%	~60%

TABLE 4.1 — CLINICAL FEATURES OF ESTABLISHED THROMBOLYTIC AGENTS

Abbreviations: APSAC, anisoylated plasminogen-streptokinase activator complex; ICH, intracranial hemorrhage; IV, intravenous; NA, not applicable; rPA, reteplase; SK, streptokinase; TIMI, Thrombosis in Myocardial Infarction; TNKase, tenecteplase; tPA, alteplase.

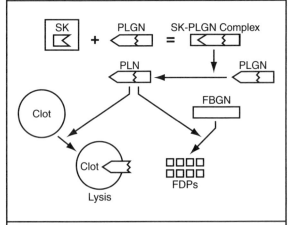
sidual plasmin continues to degrade circulating fibrinogen and other components of the clotting cascade, creating a systemic "lytic" state which increases the risk of serious bleeding and complicates the performance of invasive procedures. On a more positive note, the systemic depletion of clotting factors provides a sustained (approximately 24 hours) anticoagulant effect that reduces the risk of coronary reocclusion. Regeneration of fibrinogen and other clotting factors through hepatic synthesis occurs over the subsequent 24 to 48 hours.[9]

Streptokinase is administered intravenously at a dose of 1.5 million U given over 1 hour. Patency (TIMI 2 or 3 flow) occurs in approximately 60% of patients at 90 minutes, increasing to 80% to 90% by 24 hours. Full reperfusion, TIMI-3 flow, occurs in 35% of patients at 90 minutes, as demonstrated in the Global Use of Strategies to Open Occluded Arteries (GUSTO)-IIB angiographic substudy.[5] Numerous randomized clinical trials have demonstrated the ability of SK to reduce mortality, particularly when treatment is rendered within 6 hours of symptom onset. The landmark Gruppo Italiano per lo Studio della Streptochinasi nell'Infarcto Miocardio (GISSI) trial[10] demonstrated a 47% reduction in mortality when SK was administered within the first hour of symptom onset. Clinical benefits with SK are substantially enhanced with the addition of aspirin[3] at a dose of 160 mg to 325 mg daily, as demonstrated in the International Study of Infarct Survival (ISIS)-2 trial.[11] Antithrombotic therapy with subcutaneous heparin for patients at low risk for thromboemboli can be administered at a dose of 7,500 to 15,000 U every 12 hours, (see Chapter 13, *Acute Myocardial Infarction*), while patients at high risk for thromboemboli should receive IV heparin started 6 hours after SK therapy, when the aPTT declines to 60 seconds or less. The initial infusion rate should not exceed 1,000 U/hr. After 48 hours, options include a change to subcutaneous heparin, warfarin, or aspirin alone.[3]

Adverse reactions to SK include bleeding, hypotension, and allergic reactions. Hemorrhage occurs in approximately 5% to 10% of patients who do not undergo invasive procedures and in 15% to 20% who do. Serious bleeding occurs in 2% of patients, and intracranial hemorrhage is observed at a rate of approximately 0.5%.[3,4,9] Transient hypotension occurs commonly (in 30% to 50% of patients) particularly when the SK infusion exceeds 750,000 Units over 30 minutes. Because SK is a foreign protein, allergic reactions can and do occur in 2% to 5% of patients. Anaphylaxis, however, is rare (<0.3%).[9] Readministration of SK is not recommended between 5 days and 1 to 2 years of initial use or after recent streptococcal infection, because of the high incidence of neutralizing antibodies, leading to reduced fibrinolytic activity or allergic reactions.[9]

Anistreplase

Anisoylated plasminogen-streptokinase activator complex (APSAC), also known as anistreplase, is a stoichiometric complex containing a 1:1 ratio of SK and human blood-derived lys-plasminogen to which a para-anisoyl group has been added to "mask" the active enzymatic site. When reconstituted, APSAC deanisoylates within 30 minutes to form SK-plasminogen activator, which itself degrades to SK and plasminogen, leading to a short (30-minute) shelf life.

Anistreplase is administered as a 30 U bolus given over 5 minutes, which corresponds approximately to 1.1 million U of SK. In the circulation, gradual hydrolysis of the anisoyl group exposes the catalytic site of the complex, leading to generation of plasmin from plasminogen (Figure 4.5). The circulating half-life is approximately 90 minutes. The inactive, acyl form of the drug is thought to attenuate the generation of bradykinin, largely responsible for the hypotension seen with SK.[12] Patency rates after anistreplase are slightly higher than with SK, in the range of 75%, with full perfusion (TIMI grade 3) in approximately 50% of patients. Several large randomized trials have demonstrated reduction in mortality, improvement in left ventricular ejection fraction, and reduction in infarct size with anistreplase.[12]

The largest comparative mortality trial, ISIS-3,[13] demonstrated similar mortality outcomes for SK and anistreplase. Adverse reactions, such as bleeding, hypotension, and allergic reactions occur with similar frequency to those following SK administration. The recommendations for the conjunctive administration of aspirin and heparin parallel those for SK.

Third Generation Fibrinolytics

Novel plasminogen activators have been designed with one or more of the following properties:
- Enhanced fibrin specificity
- A prolonged half-life, permitting bolus administration
- Resistance to natural inhibitors such as PAI-1.

Reteplase (rPA), tenecteplase (TNK-tPA), lanoteplase, saruplase (single-chain urokinase plasminogen activator), and staphylokinase all represent third generation fibrinolytic agents (Tables 4.1 and 4.2).[14]

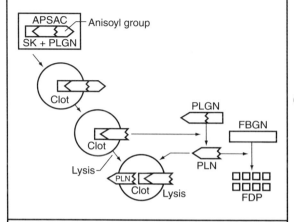

FIGURE 4.5 — MECHANISM OF ACTION OF ANISTREPLASE

Abbreviations: APSAC, anisoylated plasminogen-streptokinase activator complex; FBGN, fibrinogen; FDP, fibrinogen degradation product; PLGN, plasminogen; PLN, plasmin; SK, streptokinase.

■ **Reteplase**

Reteplase is a deletion mutant of tPA in which the finger and epidermal growth factor (EGF) domains and kringle 1 regions have been deleted, as have the carbohydrate side chains. Plasma clearance is prolonged to 18 minutes, due to reduced hepatic receptor binding and the lack of carbohydrate groups. Fibrin specificity is reduced because of the deletion of the finger domain. Reteplase is administered as two 10 MU boluses 30 minutes apart. In two large randomized trials, reteplase produced similar mortality results to SK in the International Joint Efficiency Comparison of Thrombolytics (INJECT) trial[15] and no benefit over alteplase in the GUSTO-III trial.[16] There is evidence that reteplase is associated with a higher incidence of reocclusion than alteplase, due to decreased fibrin specificity and greater platelet activation. Potent antiplatelet agents such as GPIIb/IIIa receptor antagonists may enhance the effectiveness of rPA.[17,18] The GUSTO V trial demon-

53

Feature	Lanoteplase	Staphylokinase	Saruplase
TABLE 4.2 — CLINICAL FEATURES OF NEWLY DEVELOPED FIBRINOLYTIC AGENTS			
Method of administration	Bolus	2 boluses	1-hr IV
Dose	120 KU/kg	15 + 15 mg	20-mg bolus; 60 mg over 1 hr
Half-life (min)	23	6	9
Action	Direct	Indirect	Direct
Fibrin specificity	+	++++	+
Antigenicity	NA	+	NA
PAI-1 resistance	NA	NA	+
Full perfusion (TIMI grade 3)			
60 min	47%	68%	—
90 min	57%	68%	—
Patency (TIMI grade 2/3)			
60 min	—	84%	76%
90 min	83%	84%	80%
Abbreviations: PAI-1, plasminogen-activator inhibitor-1; TIMI, Thrombolysis in Myocardial Infarction.			

strated similar 30-day mortality rates for full dose rPA and half-dose rPA combined with abciximab (5.9% and 5.6%, respectively); however, reinfarction and urgent revascularization occurred less often with combination therapy.[27] Intracranial hemorrhage rates were particularly high for patients over the age of 75, suggesting that this combination (at least with the doses given) may not be optimal for all patients with acute myocardial infarction MI) (Figure 4.6).

■ **Tenecteplase**

Tenecteplase is a genetically engineered point and deletion mutant of tPA. The amino acid substitutions and altered glycosylation sites result in a 4-fold reduction in plasma clearance, a 14-fold increased fibrin specificity, and an 80-fold greater resistance to inactivation by PAI-1.[17] The long plasma half-life permits a single push bolus (Table 4.2). Angiographic observations derived from the TIMI 10A and 10B trials suggested that tenecteplase achieved faster and more complete reperfusion than alteplase;[18] however, the recently reported Assessment of the Safety and Efficacy of a New Thrombolytic (ASSENT)-2 trial comparing TNK-tPA and alteplase in 16,000 patients demonstrated equivalent outcomes, with a lower risk of bleeding associated with TNK-tPA.[19]

The ASSENT 3[28] trial has further characterized the benefits of tenecteplase in acute MI. In this trial, 6095 patients were randomly assigned to full dose TNK-tPA with weight-adjusted unfractionated heparin,[3] TNK-tPA with enoxaparin, or reduced-dose tenecteplase with abciximab. Mortality at 30 days was similar among the three treatment groups (6.6%, 5.4%, and 6%, respectively), with a trend toward lower mortality in the TNK-tPA plus enoxaparin group (Figure 4.6). There were significantly fewer cumulative efficacy end points in the enoxaparin and abciximab groups (11.4% and 11.1%) than in the unfractionated heparin group (15.4%). Similar to observations made in GUSTO V, intracranial hemorrhage occurred more frequently in patients over the age of 75 who received the combination of a fibrinolytic agent and abciximab.

These data suggest that enhanced speed and extent of thrombolysis is achievable by combining more effective antiplatelet therapy with reduced doses of fibrinolytic drugs.

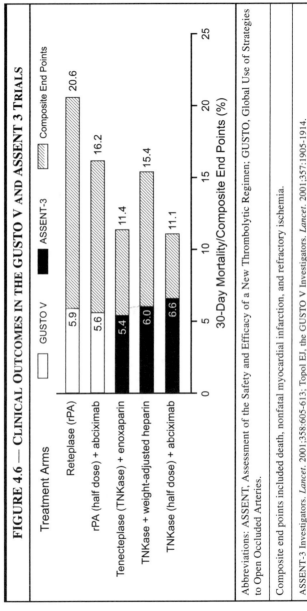

FIGURE 4.6 — CLINICAL OUTCOMES IN THE GUSTO V AND ASSENT 3 TRIALS

Legend: GUSTO V | ASSENT-3 | Composite End Points

Treatment Arms

Reteplase (rPA) — 5.9, 20.6

rPA (half dose) + abciximab — 5.6, 16.2

Tenecteplase (TNKase) + enoxaparin — 5.4, 11.4

TNKase + weight-adjusted heparin — 6.0, 15.4

TNKase (half dose) + abciximab — 6.6, 11.1

30-Day Mortality/Composite End Points (%)

Abbreviations: ASSENT, Assessment of the Safety and Efficacy of a New Thrombolytic Regimen; GUSTO, Global Use of Strategies to Open Occluded Arteries.

Composite end points included death, nonfatal myocardial infarction, and refractory ischemia.

ASSENT-3 Investigators. *Lancet.* 2001;358:605-613; Topol EJ, the GUSTO V Investigators. *Lancet.* 2001;357:1905-1914.

They also show that benefits and risks of combined pharmacotherapy vary in patient subgroups. Accordingly, more information is needed before this particular combination can be recommended routinely for patients with acute ST-elevation MI. On the other hand, combining tPA or TNK-tPA with anticoagulants like enoxaparin appears to be a promising reperfusion regimen that also offers ease of administration.

■ Lanoteplase

Lanoteplase is a deletion and "point" mutant of wild-type tPA, in which the glycosylation sites in kringle 1 have been modified and the EGF and finger domains have been removed. It has a prolonged half-life of 37 minutes, reduced fibrin affinity, and improved thrombolytic efficacy in animal models (Table 4.2).[17] TIMI-3 flow rates at 60 and 90 minutes compare favorably with alteplase. However, a large randomized trial, Intravenous nPA Treatment of Infarcting Myocardium Early II (InTIME-2), while demonstrating similar mortality outcomes to accelerated tPA, also revealed a higher rate of intracranial hemorrhage in patients receiving lanoteplase. Further development of the agent has not taken place.

■ Saruplase

Saruplase, also known as single-chain urokinase plasminogen activator or prourokinase, is a naturally occurring glycoprotein prodrug that is rapidly converted into urokinase by plasmin but has some intrinsic plasminogen activating properties as well.[20] The half-life is very short, in the range of 7 to 8 minutes (Table 4.2). Saruplase produces a systemic "lytic" state as demonstrated by decreases in fibrinogen and alpha$_2$-antiplasmin and increased fibrinogen degradation products.[17,21,22] Several trials have revealed similar patency rates between saruplase and a 3-hour infusion regimen of tPA [22] and slightly lower mortality than with SK but at a cost of increased intracranial hemorrhage.[23] Future modifications of the compound include chimeric variants consisting of the two kringle domains of tPA and the serine protease domain of saruplase, as well as chemical modification of saruplase with cross-linking with antifibrin and antiplatelet antibodies, with the aim of increasing drug concentration at the site of thrombus formation.[17]

- **Staphylokinase**

Staphylokinase, a 136-amino acid protein produced naturally by strains of *Staphylococcus aureus*, is currently synthesized using recombinant techniques. Like SK, it must form a stoichiometric 1:1 complex with plasminogen, which must then be activated by plasminogen activators. This agent has high fibrin specificity and a unique mechanism of action.[17,24] Like SK, staphylokinase triggers antibodies in most patients within 2 weeks after initial administration. Allergic reactions were not reported in the early clinical trials, possibly due to the low molecular weight of the staphylokinase molecule. Although several small, comparative trials with tPA were promising,[25] large-scale randomized trials will be needed to determine its overall clinical potential and safety.

Goals for Future Development of Fibrinolytic Agents

Strategies to achieve optimal outcomes with fibrinolytic therapy include:
- Earlier administration
- Better and more easily administered compounds
- Better conjunctive antithrombotic therapies, such as low molecular weight heparin, direct antithrombins, and/or GPIIb/IIIa receptor antagonists
- Reduced reocclusion and reinfarction rates
- Better selection of patients for facilitated revascularization
- Reduced reperfusion damage through the use of microcirculatory "protective" agents, such as neutrophil chemotaxis or adhesion antagonists.

Long-term approaches to treatment will include:
- Plaque stabilizing agents
- Lipid-modifying agents
- Inflammatory response modulating agents

- Angiotensin-converting enzyme inhibitors or angiotensin receptor blockers to attenuate left ventricular remodeling
- Defined pharmacologic approaches to prevent late sudden death.[14]

Further refinement of currently available fibrinolytics either alone or in combination with anticoagulants and platelet antagonists will be required as we maximize treatments for the new millennium.

4

REFERENCES

1. Stump DC, Collen D. The Fibrinolytic System: Implications for Thrombolytic Therapy. In: Califf R, Mark D, Wagner G, ed. *Acute Coronary Care in the Thrombolytic Era*. Chicago, Ill: Year Book Medical Publishers, Inc; 1988.

2. Collen D, Verstraete M. Alpha$_2$-antiplasmin consumption and fibrinogen breakdown during thrombolytic therapy. *Thromb Res*. 1979; 14:631-639.

3. Ryan TJ, Antman EM, Brooks NH, et al. 1999 update: ACC/AHA guidelines for the management of patients with acute myocardial infarction. A report of the American College of Cardiology/American Heart Association Task Force on Practice Guidelines (Committee on Management of Acute Myocardial Infarction). *J Am Coll Cardiol*. 1999;34:890-911.

4. The GUSTO Investigators. An international randomized trial comparing four thrombolytic strategies for acute myocardial infarction. *N Engl J Med*. 1993;329:673-682.

5. The GUSTO Angiographic Investigators. The effects of tissue plasminogen activator, streptokinase, or both on coronary-artery patency, ventricular function, and survival after acute myocardial infarction (published correction appears in *N Engl J Med*. 1994;330:516.). *N Engl J Med*. 1993;329:1615-1622.

6. Antman EM, Giugliano RP, Gibson CM, et al for the TIMI 14 Investigators. Abciximab facilitates the rate and extent of thrombolysis: results of the thrombolysis in myocardial infarction (TIMI)-14 trial. *Circulation*. 1999;99:2720-2732.

7. Brener S. Presentation of INTRO-AMI Data. AHA Scientific Sessions, November 1999.

8. Sherry S. Personal reflections on the development of thrombolytic therapy and its application to acute coronary thrombosis. *Am Heart J*. 1981;102:1134-1138.

9. Anderson J, Smith B. Streptokinase in acute myocardial infarction. In: Anderson J, ed. *Modern Management of Myocardial Infarction in the Community Hospital.* Marcel Dekker, NY; 1991:187-215.

10. Gruppo Italiano per lo Studio della Streptochinasi nell'Infarto Miocardico (GISSI). Effectiveness of intravenous thrombolytic treatment in acute myocardial infarction. *Lancet.* 1986;1:397-402.

11. ISIS-2 (Second International Study of Infarct Survival) Collaborative Group. Randomised trial of intravenous streptokinase, oral aspirin, both, or neither among 17,187 cases of suspected acute myocardial infarction: ISIS-2. *Lancet.* 1988;2:349-360.

12. Anderson, J. Review of anistreplase (APSAC) for acute myocardial infarction. In: Anderson J, ed. *Modern Management of Myocardial Infarction in the Community Hospital.* Marcel Dekker, NY, 1991:149-185.

13. ISIS-3 (Third International Study of Infarct Survival) Collaborative Group. A randomised comparison of streptokinase vs tissue plasminogen activator vs anistreplase and of aspirin plus heparin vs aspirin alone among 41,299 cases of suspected acute myocardial infarction: ISIS-3. *Lancet.* 1992;339:753-770.

14. White HD, Van de Werf FJ. Thrombolysis for acute myocardial infarction. *Circulation.* 1998;97:1632-1646.

15. International Joint Efficacy Comparison of Thrombolytics. Randomised, double-blind comparison of reteplase double-bolus administration with streptokinase in acute myocardial infarction (INJECT): trial to investigate equivalence. *Lancet.* 1995;346:329-336.

16. The Global Use of Strategies to Open Occluded Coronary Arteries (GUSTO III) Investigators. A comparison of reteplase with alteplase for acute myocardial infarction. *N Engl J Med.* 1997;337:1118-1123.

17. Ross AM. New plasminogen activators: a clinical review. *Clin Cardiol.* 1999;22:165-171.

18. The SPEED Study Group. Trial of abciximab with and without low-dose reteplase for acute myocardial infarction. Strategies for Patency Enhancement in the Emergency Department (SPEED) Group. *Circulation.* 2000;101:2788-2794.

19. Cannon CP, Gibson MC, McCabe CH. TNK-tissue plasminogen activator compared with front-loaded alteplase in acute myocardial infarction: results of the TIMI 10B trial. *Circulation.* 1998;98:2805-2814.

20. Presentation of ASSENT-2 data at the AHA Meeting, November 1999, Atlanta, GA.

21. de Munk GAW, Ryken DC. Fibrinolytic properties of single-chain urokinase-type plasminogen activator (pro-urokinase). *Fibrinolysis.* 1990;4:1-9.

22. PRIMI Trial Study Group. Randomised double-blind trial of recombinant pro-urokinase against streptokinase in acute myocardial infarction. *Lancet.* 1989;1:863-868.

23. Bar FW, Meyer J, Vermeer F, et al for the SESAM Study Group. Comparison of saruplase and alteplase in acute myocardial infarction. The Study in Europe with Saruplase and Alteplase in Myocardial Infarction. *Am J Cardiol.* 1997;79:727-732.

24. Tebbe U, Michels R, Adgey J, et al for the Comparison Trial of Saruplase and Streptokinase (COMPASS) Investigators. Randomized, double-blind study comparing saruplase with streptokinase therapy in acute myocardial infarction: the COMPASS equivalence trial. *J Am Coll Cardiol.* 1998;31:487-493.

25. Collen D, Lijnen HR. Staphylokinase, a fibrin-specific plasminogen activator with therapeutic potential? *Blood.* 1994;84:680-686.

26. Vanderschueren S, Dens J, Kerdsinchai P, et al. Randomized coronary patency trial of double-bolus recombinant staphylokinase versus front-loaded alteplase in acute myocardial infarction. *Am Heart J.* 1997;134:213-219.

27. Topol EJ, The GUSTO V Investigators. Reperfusion therapy for acute myocardial infarction with fibrinolytic therapy or combination reduced fibrinolytic therapy and platelet glycoprotein IIb/IIIa inhibition: the GUSTO V randomised trial. *Lancet.* 2001;357:1905-1914.

28. The Assessment of the Safety and Efficacy of a New Thrombolytic Regimen (ASSENT)-3 Investigators. Efficacy and safety of tenecteplase in combination with enoxaparin, abciximab, or unfractionated heparin: the ASSENT-3 randomised trial in acute myocardial infarction. *Lancet.* 2001;358:605-613.

5   Aspirin

The development of oral and intravenous pharmacologic agents that selectively attenuate platelet function for clinical use in patients with atherosclerotic vascular disease has contributed greatly to improved outcomes worldwide.

Aspirin, considered the prototypic platelet antagonist, has been available for over a century and currently represents a mainstay both in the prevention and treatment of vascular events that include stroke, myocardial infarction, and sudden death.

Mechanism of Action

Aspirin irreversibly acetylates cyclooxygenase (COX), impairing prostaglandin metabolism and thromboxane A_2 (TXA_2) synthesis. As a result, platelet aggregation in response to collagen, adenosine diphosphate (ADP), thrombin (in low concentrations), and TXA_2 is inhibited.[1,2]

Because aspirin more selectively inhibits COX-1 activity (found predominantly in platelets) than COX-2 activity (expressed in tissues following an inflammatory stimuli), its ability to prevent platelet aggregation is seen at relatively low doses, compared with the drug's potential anti-inflammatory effects, which require much higher doses.[3] As a result, the benefit derived from aspirin therapy more than likely represents an antithrombotic effect.

Several alternative mechanisms of platelet inhibition by aspirin have been proposed:

- Aspirin facilitates the inhibition of platelet activation by neutrophils
- Inhibition of prostacyclin synthesis in endothelial cells enhances nitric oxide production.

In addition, aspirin may prevent the progression of atherosclerosis by protecting low-density lipoprotein (LDL) cholesterol from oxidation and scavenging hydroxyl radicals.

Pharmacokinetics

Following oral ingestion, aspirin is rapidly absorbed in the proximal gastrointestinal (GI) tract (stomach, duodenum), achieving peak serum levels within 15 to 20 minutes and platelet inhibition within 40 to 60 minutes. As would be expected, enteric-coated preparations are less well absorbed, causing a delay in peak serum levels and platelet inhibition to 60 and 90 minutes, respectively. The antiplatelet effect occurs even before acetylsalicylic acid is detectable in peripheral blood, owing of platelet exposure in the portal circulation.

The plasma concentration of aspirin decays rapidly with a circulating half-life of approximately 20 minutes. Despite the drug's rapid clearance, platelet inhibition persists for the platelet's life span (7 ± 2 days) due to aspirin's irreversible inactivation of COX-1. Because 10% of circulating platelets are replaced every 24 hours, platelet activity (bleeding time, primary hemostasis) returns toward normal (≥50% activity) within 5 to 6 days of the last aspirin dose.[4] A single dose of 100 mg aspirin effectively reduces the production of TXA_2 in normal individuals.

Adverse Effects

The adverse-effect profile of aspirin in general and its associated risk for major hemorrhage in particular is determined largely by:

- Dose
- Duration of administration
- Associated structural (peptic ulcer disease, *Helicobacter pylori* infection) and hemostatic (inherited, acquired) abnormalities
- Concomitant use of other antithrombotic agents.

Thus aspirin is usually well tolerated when given in low doses (≤325 mg) for brief periods of time (6 to 8 weeks) to patients at low risk for bleeding complications. Unfortunately, a majority of conditions for which aspirin is considered the standard of care persist over time (eg, atherosclerotic vascular disease) necessitating prolonged periods of exposure. For this reason, aspirin, like all antithrombotic drugs that can also compromise hemostatic capacity, should only be given after a comprehensive evaluation of an individual patient's thrombotic and hemorrhagic risk has been established.

Enteric coating of aspirin has *not* been shown to reduce the likelihood of adverse effects involving the GI tract. Patients with gastric erosions or peptic ulcer disease who require treatment with aspirin should concomitantly receive a proton pump inhibitor to minimize the risk of hemorrhage.[5]

The impact of aspirin use on the hemodynamic properties of angiotensin-converting enzyme (ACE) inhibitors is a subject of considerable clinical relevance. Because COX-1 participates in prostaglandin production, which in turn, influences vascular tone, drugs with preferential COX-1 activity would be expected to interact with ACE inhibitors to a greater extent than COX-2 antagonists. The available evidence, derived from retrospective analyses, suggests that the antihypertensive and hemodynamic benefits are attenuated when doses of aspirin in excess of 100 mg are administered daily. This effect may be particularly important in patients with poor ventricular performance and clinical heart failure. In these settings, alternative vascular/hemodynamic (eg, angiotensin II receptor antagonist) and antithrombotic (eg, clopidogrel) therapies should be considered.

The interaction of aspirin and ACE inhibitors does not influence short-term outcome following acute myocardial infarction (MI),[6] but must be considered with prolonged coadministration, particularly in patients with poor left ventricular function and moderate to severe congestive heart failure. In this setting, the aspirin dose should be limited to 100 mg or less.

Clinical Efficacy

Aspirin's beneficial effect is determined largely by the absolute risk of vascular events. Patients at low risk (healthy individuals without predisposing risk factors for vascular disease) derive minimal benefit, while those at high risk (unstable angina, prior MI, stroke) derive considerable benefit (Figure 5.1).[7] A risk-based approach to aspirin administration is recommended to avoid subjecting individuals

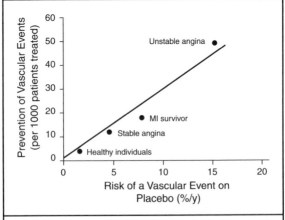

FIGURE 5.1 — BENEFITS OF ASPIRIN ADMINISTRATION BASED ON RISK FOR VASCULAR EVENTS

The risk-benefit ratio of aspirin administration is determined by a patient's overall likelihood of experiencing a vascular event. Patients at greatest risk derive the greatest benefit from daily treatment.

Chest. 2001;119:49S.

who are unlikely to benefit from aspirin administration to its potential adverse effects (Table 5.1).

Primary Prevention

Aspirin has been evaluated in three primary prevention trials involving over 30,000 healthy individuals.[8-10] A fourth trial confirmed the benefit of low-dose aspirin in patients with hypertension.[11] The Women's Health Initiative is evaluating the effects of low-dose aspirin prophylaxis (100 mg every other day) in 40,000 healthy women.

Considered collectively, the data show convincingly that aspirin reduces the likelihood of MI but at a cost of increased risk for hemorrhagic complications, including stroke. With increasing patient risk (for thrombotic events), additional benefit is gained, improving net clinical benefit.

TABLE 5.1 — RECOMMENDATIONS FOR ASPIRIN ADMINISTRATION	
Clinical Setting	**Recommendation**
Primary prevention	Not indicated unless risk factors*
Treatment of acute MI, unstable angina, ischemic stroke	Risk factors*: 75-162.5 mg/d; initial therapy: 162.5-325 mg; subsequent dose: 75-162.5 mg/d
Secondary prevention: chronic stable angina, MI, stroke, TIA	Daily therapy 75-325 mg

Abbreviations: MI, myocardial infarction; TIA, transient ischemic attack.

* Risk factors: men and women >50 years of age who have at least one major risk factor for coronary artery disease (cigarette smoking, hypertension, diabetes mellitus, high cholesterol level, history of parental myocardial infarction).

Secondary Prevention

The Antiplatelet Trialists' Collaboration provides firm evidence in support of aspirin's ability to prevent vascular events, including nonfatal MI, nonfatal stroke, and vascular death in a wide range of high-risk patient groups. In high-risk patients as a whole, antiplatelet therapy (predominantly with aspirin) reduces nonfatal MI by approximately one third, nonfatal stroke by one third, and vascular death by nearly one quarter (Figure 5.2).[12]

Patients with prior aspirin use who experience an acute coronary syndrome "aspirin failures" are at particularly high risk for MI and death over the ensuing weeks to months, suggesting a stimulus for thrombosis that overcomes the modest inhibitory potential of aspirin. Combination therapy to include a platelet adenosine diphosphate (ADP) antagonist (eg, clopidogrel) makes sound clinical sense in these individuals (Figure 5.3).[13]

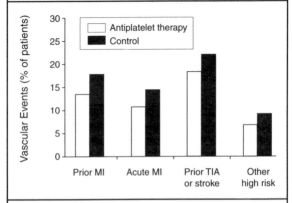

FIGURE 5.2 — REDUCED VASCULAR EVENT RATES IN HIGH-RISK PATIENTS WITH ANTIPLATELET THERAPY

Antiplatelet therapy, predominately with aspirin, significantly reduces vascular-event rates (fatal/nonfatal myocardial infarction [MI], transient ischemic attack [TIA], stroke, cardiovascular death) in high-risk patients. $P <0.00001$.

The Antiplatelet Trialists' Collaboration. *Br Med J.* 1994;308:81-106.

Dosing

Aspirin dose varied widely in the Antiplatelet Trialists' Collaboration overview, ranging from 75 mg to 1500 mg daily; however, indirect comparisons failed to identify differences that favored higher over lower doses (Table 5.2). Accordingly, a maintenance dose of 75 mg to 100 mg daily may be adequate in a majority of high-risk patients. A higher dose (160 mg to 325 mg) is recommended when treatment is first being initiated to rapidly provide antiplatelet effects.

Coronary Artery Bypass Grafting

Patients undergoing coronary artery bypass surgery are unique for several reasons. First, a majority of patients have advanced coronary atherosclerosis. Second, many individu-

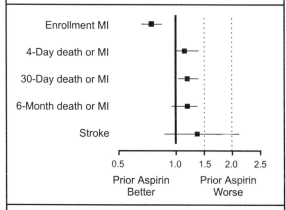

FIGURE 5.3 — ASSOCIATION BETWEEN PRIOR ASPIRIN USE AND CLINICAL OUTCOMES AT 30 DAYS

Abbreviation: MI, myocardial infarction.

Odds ratios and 95% confidence intervals for the association between prior aspirin use and clinical outcomes at 30 days.

Alexander JH, et al. *Am J Cardiol.* 1999;83:1147-51.

TABLE 5.2 — INDIRECT COMPARISON OF ASPIRIN DOSE AND REDUCTION IN VASCULAR EVENTS

Aspirin Dose (mg/d)	Clinical Trials (n)	Patients (n)	Event Reduction (%)
500-1500	30	18,471	21.4
160-325	12	23,670	28.3
75	4	5,012	29.7

als have concomitant peripheral vascular and cerebrovascular disease. Last, new vascular conduits (bypass grafts) provide an additional nidus for atherothrombosis. Over the years, in excess of 20 clinical trials have been conducted to determine the effectiveness of antiplatelet therapy in preventing early ($\leq$10 days) and late (6 to 12 months) saphenous vein graft occlusion. Ten of the trials investigated aspirin in doses ranging from 100 mg to 975 mg daily. Several also evaluated patients receiving internal mammary coronary bypass grafts.[14-19]

Considered collectively, and aided by the Antiplatelet Trialists' Collaboration overview, the data reveal improved saphenous vein graft patency with aspirin administration. Although a direct benefit on internal mammary bypass grafts has not been established, treatment is recommended given the common coexistence of vascular disease (and the risk of thrombotic events). A majority of evidence supporting the use of aspirin after bypass grafting is based on clinical trials using a dose of at least 325 mg daily. Accordingly, the benefit derived from lower doses is not entirely clear. Patients unable to take aspirin should be given clopidogrel 300 mg (loading dose) 6 hours after surgery followed by 75 mg daily.

Transient Ischemic Attacks/Stroke

The International Stroke Trial[20] and the Chinese Acute Stroke Trial[21] evaluated the efficacy and safety of aspirin given in a daily dose of 300 mg and 160 mg, respectively, in nearly 40,000 patients with acute ischemic stroke. Treatment was initiated within 48 hours of symptom onset and continued for 2 to 4 weeks. The combined results suggest an absolute benefit of 10 fewer deaths or nonfatal strokes per 1000 patients in the first month of treatment. The risk of hemorrhagic stroke was also increased (two excess events per 1000 patients).

Long-term aspirin administration reduces the likelihood of stroke (and other vascular events) in patients with transient ischemic attacks and completed minor strokes.[22] Although there is an ongoing debate within the neurology community concerning the optimal daily dose, 75 mg to 325 mg is considered an acceptable range.

The combination of aspirin (25 mg) and extended-release dipyridamole (200 mg bid) is more effective than aspirin alone for the prevention of stroke. Patients unable to take aspirin should be treated with clopidogrel (75 mg daily).

Percutaneous Coronary Intervention

Percutaneous coronary intervention (PCI), including standard balloon angioplasty, rotational atherectomy, and laser angioplasty, with or without stent placement, is associated with vascular injury, atheromatous plaque disruption, platelet activation, and at times, coronary thromboembolism. Several studies performed over the past decade have documented reduced periprocedural complications, including thrombus formation, abrupt closure, and MI, with antiplatelet therapy given prior to PCI (relative risk reduction, 60%).[23,24]

The current recommendations for PCI include aspirin (80 to 325 mg) pretreatment followed by long-term administration (80 to 325 mg daily) for secondary prevention of cardiovascular events; for patients unable to tolerate aspirin, pretreatment with clopidogrel (300 mg) followed by 75 mg daily is suggested.

The Importance of Aspirin Resistance

Aspirin's ability to inhibit platelet aggregation is discordant and upward of 30% of individuals either are nonresponders or exhibit a paradoxical increase in platelet aggregation and activation following high-dose (325 mg) administration.

Nearly a century ago, Duke reported that patients with anemia and thrombocytopenia experienced a shortening of their bleeding time following transfusion, raising the possibility that platelet behavior is influenced directly by erythrocytes.[25] In vitro, erythrocytes augment platelet activation through several mechanisms, including:
- Physical interactions
- Adenosine diphosphate-mediated agonists
- Facilitated TXA_2 production.

The interplay between erythrocytes and platelets has important clinical implications with regard to aspirin dosing. Low-dose aspirin (80 mg) inhibits TXA_2 production; however, the relationship between TXA_2 concentration and platelet activation is nonlinear, suggesting one or more alternative pathways of platelet activation that includes thrombin, serotonin, and platelet-activating factor. Erythrocytes can activate platelets in the presence of low-dose aspirin, but Santos and colleagues have shown that the acute administration of higher doses (500 mg) suppresses residual red blood cell–facilitated platelet function.[26]

Thromboxane A_2, a potent platelet agonist, must be suppressed by 90% or more for complete inhibition. Aspirin's ability to reduce COX activity varies considerably among individuals and, in addition, atherosclerosis is associated with increased tissue level expression due to cytokine-mediated induction. Lastly, genetic polymorphisms and resulting gene expression of COX and thromboxane synthase could limit aspirin effectiveness (Figure 5.4).[27]

Clinical Impact of Aspirin Resistance and Failures

Despite its proven benefit, aspirin does have inherent limitations. A critical review of the existing literature reveals a sizable proportion of events in patients receiving aspirin. If one were to adopt a "half empty" view toward aspirin, between 60% and 70% of patients experience MI, stroke, or cardiovascular death during periods of treatment (Table 5.3).

Summary

Aspirin is a time-tested platelet antagonist that is widely available, inexpensive, and well tolerated, even with long-term administration.[28] High-risk patients enjoy the greatest overall benefit, with a relative reduction in major vascular-event rates approaching 25% to 30%. The discordant effects of aspirin on platelet aggregation, aspirin "resistance," aspirin failures, and the added benefit of combined pharmacotherapy must be investigated through large-scale clinical trials.

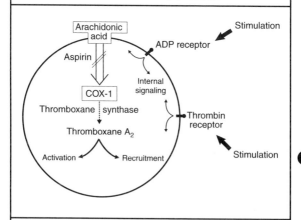
REFERENCES

1. Roth GJ, Majerus PW. The mechanism of the effect of aspirin on human platelets. I. Acetylation of a particulate fraction protein. *J Clin Invest*. 1975;56:624-632.

2. Burch JW, Stanford N, Majerus PW. Inhibition of platelet prostaglandin synthetase by oral aspirin. *J Clin Invest*. 1978;61:314-319.

3. Patrono C. Aspirin as an antiplatelet drug. *N Engl J Med*. 1994;330:1287-1294.

4. O'Brien JR. Effects of salicylates on human platelets. *Lancet*. 1968;1:779-783.

5. Hawkey CJ, Karrasch JA, Szczepañski L, et al. Omeprazole compared with misoprostol for ulcers associated with nonsteroidal anti-inflammatory drugs. Omeprazole versus Misprostol for NSAID-induced Ulcer Management (OMNIUM) Study Group. *N Engl J Med*. 1998;338:727-734.

TABLE 5.3 — THE STRENGTHS AND WEAKNESSES OF ASPIRIN THERAPY			
Patient Group	Relative Risk Reduction (%)*	Absolute Risk Reduction (n)†	Majority of Patients Remain at Risk
Chronic stable angina	33	45	Yes
Unstable angina	39	50	Yes
Acute myocardial infarction	29	38	Yes
Post-myocardial infarction	25	36	Yes

* Effect on major vascular events.
† Per 1000 patients.

6. Latini R, Tognoni G, Maggioni AP, et al. Clinical effects of early angiotensin-converting enzyme inhibitor treatment for acute myocardial infarction are similar in the presence and absence of aspirin: systemic overview of individual data from 96,712 randomized patients. Angiotensin-converting Enzyme Inhibitor Myocardial Infarction Collaborative Group. *J Am Coll Cardiol.* 2000;35:1801-1807.

7. Awtry EH, Loscalzo J. Aspirin. *Circulation.* 2000;101:1206-1218.

8. Steering Committee of the Physicians' Health Study Research Group. Final report on the aspirin component of the ongoing Physicians' Health Study. *N Engl J Med.* 1989;321:129-135.

9. The Medical Research Council's General Practice Research Framework. Thrombosis prevention trial: randomized trial of low intensity oral anticoagulation with warfarin and low-dose aspirin in the primary prevention of ischaemic heart disease in men at increased risk. *Lancet.* 1998;351:233-241.

10. Peto R, Gray R, Collins R, et al. Randomised trial of prophylactic daily aspirin in British male doctors. *Br Med J.* 1988;926:313-316.

11. Hansson L, Zanchetti A, Carruthers SG, et al. Effects of intensive blood-pressure lowering and low-dose aspirin in patients with hypertension: principal results of the Hypertension Optimal Treatment (HOT) randomised trial. HOT Study Group. *Lancet.* 1998;351:1755-1762.

12. Antiplatelet Trialists' Collaboration. Collaborative overview of randomised trials of antiplatelet therapy—I: Prevention of death, myocardial infarction, and stroke by prolonged antiplatelet therapy in various categories of patients. *BMJ.* 1994:308;81-106.

13. Alexander JH, Harrington RA, Tuttle RH, et al. Prior aspirin use predicts worse outcomes in patients with non-ST elevation acute coronary syndromes. PURSUIT Investigators. Platelet IIb/IIIa in Unstable angina: Receptor Suppression Using Integrilin Therapy. *Am J Cardiol.* 1999;83:1147-1151.

14. Lorenz RL, Schacky CV, Weber M, et al. Improved aortocoronary bypass patency by low-dose aspirin (100 mg daily). Effects of platelet aggregation and thromboxane formation. *Lancet.* 1984;1:1261-1264.

15. Hockings BE, Ireland MA, Gotch-Martin KF, Taylor RR. Placebo-controlled trial of enteric coated aspirin in coronary bypass graft patients. Effect on graft patency. *Med J Aust.* 1993;159:376-378.

16. Goldman S, Copeland J, Moritz T, et al. Improvement in early saphenous vein graft patency after coronary artery bypass surgery with antiplatelet therapy: results of a Veterans Administration Cooperative Study. *Circulation.* 1988;77:1324-1332.

5

17. Goldman S, Copeland J, Moritz T, et al. Internal mammary artery and saphenous vein graft patency. Effects of aspirin. *Circulation*. 1990;82(suppl):IV237-IV242.

18. van der Meer J, Brutel de la Riviere A, van Gilst WH, et al. Effects of low-dose aspirin (50 mg/day), low dose aspirin plus dipyridamole, and oral anticoagulant agents after internal mammary artery bypass grafting: patency and clinical outcome at 1 year. CABADAS Researcj Group of the Interuniversity Cardiology Institute of The Netherlands. Prevention of Coronary Artery Bypass Graft Occlusion by Aspirin, Dipyridamole and Acenocoumarol/Phenprocoumon Study. *J Am Coll Cardiol*. 1994;24:1181-1188.

19. Brown BG, Cukingnan RA, De Rouen T, et al. Improved graft patency in patients treated with platelet-inhibiting therapy after coronary bypass surgery. *Circulation*. 1985;72:138-146.

20. International Stroke Trial Collaborative Group. The International Stroke Trial (IST): a randomised trial of aspirin, subcutaneous heparin, both, or neither among 19,435 patients with acute ischaemic stroke. *Lancet*. 1997;349:1569-1581.

21. CAST (Chinese Acute Stroke Trial) Collaborative Group. CAST: randomised placebo-controlled trial of early aspirin use in 20,000 patients with acute ischaemic stroke. *Lancet*. 1997;349:1641-1649.

22. The SALT Collaborative Group. Swedish Aspirin Low-Dose Trial (SALT) of 75 mg aspirin as secondary prophylaxis after cerebrovascular ischaemic events. *Lancet*. 1991;338:1345-1349.

23. Barnathan ES, Schwartz JS, Taylor L, et al. Aspirin and dipyridamole in the prevention of acute coronary thrombosis complicating coronary angioplasty. *Circulation*. 1987;76:125-134.

24. Schwartz L, Bourassa MG, Lesperance J, et al. Aspirin and dipyridamole in the prevention of restenosis after percutaneous transluminal coronary angioplasty. *N Engl J Med*. 1988;318:1714-1719.

25. Duke WW. The relation of blood platelets to hemorrhagic disease. *JAMA*. 1983;250:1201-1209.

26. Santos MT, Valles J, Aznar J, Marcus AJ, Broekman MJ, Safier LB. Prothrombotic effects of erythrocytes on platelet reactivity. Reduction by aspirin. *Circulation*. 1997;95:63-68.

27. Nair GV, Davis CJ, McKenzie ME, Lowry DR, Serebruany VL. Aspirin in patients with coronary artery disease: Is it Simply Irresistable? *J Thromb Thrombolysis*. 2001;11:117-126.

28. Sixth American College of Chest Physicians. Conference on antithrombotic therapy. *Chest*. 2001;119(suppl 1):1S-370S.

76

6   Ticlopidine

Ticlopidine (Ticlid) is a thienopyridine derivative that is structurally and functionally distinct from most platelet antagonists.

In Vitro Effects

In vitro, ticlopidine is a weak inhibitor of platelet aggregation. Against low concentrations of collagen, arachidonic acid, or adenosine diphosphate (ADP), ticlopidine exhibits much less antiaggregative activity than aspirin.[1]

In addition to its modest *in vitro* platelet-inhibiting properties, ticlopidine:
- Attenuates endothelial cell growth
- Increases endothelial cell–associated von Willebrand factor concentrations.[2]

Ex Vivo Effect on Platelet Function

After oral administration, ticlopidine becomes a concentration-dependent inhibitor of ADP-mediated platelet aggregation.[3,4] With standard dosing, platelet inhibition is evident within 24 to 48 hours; however, peak effects are not produced for 3 to 6 days. The platelet-inhibiting effects of ticlopidine persist for 72 hours after the drugs discontinuation and progressive decline over the next 4 to 8 days. A synergistic effect on platelet inhibition has been reported with the combined administration of aspirin and ticlopidine.[5]

Although ticlopidine has lipophilic properties that can affect the fluidity of platelet membrane lipids, there is no evidence that it directly inhibits ADP binding. Ticlopidine does inhibit fibrinogen binding but does so without inducing a quantitative change in the surface glycoprotein (GP) IIb/IIIa receptor.[6]

Nonplatelet Effects

Ticlopidine binds to erythrocyte membranes and improves cellular deformability in response to shear stress. *In vitro*, ticlopidine dose-dependently inhibits platelet-mediated neutrophil activation, and in patients undergoing hemodialysis, reduces complement-mediated leukocyte trapping within the pulmonary circulation.[7]

Pharmacokinetics

Ticlopidine is well absorbed following oral administration, with peak plasma concentrations occurring within 1 to 3 hours. It is rapidly and extensively metabolized in the liver to one or more metabolites that are responsible for the drug's platelet-inhibiting properties.

Side Effects

Approximately 10% to 15% of patients receiving ticlopidine at the recommended dosage of 250 mg twice daily (taken with food) experience side effects, the most common of which are gastrointestinal complaints and skin rash. Bleeding is relatively uncommon, but can occur. Cholestatic jaundice and hepatitis have also been reported.

Ticlopidine's hematologic side effects, including agranulocytosis, neutropenia, erythroleukemia, thrombocytopenia, and thrombotic thrombocytopenic purpura (TTP), are the most concerning and potentially life-threatening.

In an overview of 60 cases of TTP associated with ticlopidine administration, the drug had been taken for less than 1 month by 80% of patients and a normal platelet count was documented within 2 weeks of the disorders' onset.[8] A retrospective analysis of 43,322 patients undergoing coronary stenting at study sites participating in the Evaluation of Platelet GPIIb/IIIa Inhibitor for Stenting (EPISTENT) Study disclosed an incidence of 1 case per 4,814 patients treated.[9] Although an infrequent occurrence, the 0.02% incidence is noteworthy (and clinically relevant) when the estimated 0.0004% incidence in the general population is considered. Thus close monitoring of platelet counts is recommended, particularly if therapy is continued beyond 2 weeks.

The ability of ticlopidine to inhibit platelet aggregation in a dose-dependent manner, coupled with the synergistic effects observed when it is combined with aspirin, has led to a relatively large clinical experience that spans a variety of cardiovascular settings (Tables 6.1 and 6.2).

■ Coronary Artery Disease

Patients with coronary artery disease at risk for thrombotic events have been treated, some for prolonged periods of time, with ticlopidine. A majority were either intolerant or allergic to aspirin. Despite an anecdotal experience, ticlopidine's use in the primary prevention of cardiovascular events has not been studied in large-scale randomized trials.

■ Stable Angina Pectoris

Several small-scale studies of patients with stable angina pectoris have been performed, each showing reduced platelet aggregation in response to ADP, collagen, and epinephrine following ticlopidine administration.[10] Despite a change in platelet responsiveness following exercise,[11] there was no clear impact on overall exercise tolerance or ischemic response.

■ Unstable Angina

In a multicenter trial of 652 patients admitted to the hospital with a diagnosis of unstable angina, conventional therapy (β-blocker, nitrates, calcium channel antagonists) plus ticlopidine (250 mg bid) reduced the likelihood of vascular death or nonfatal myocardial infarction (MI) by nearly 50% compared with conventional therapy alone. The composite end point of fatal and nonfatal MI was reduced by over 50%.[12]

■ Myocardial Infarction

The administration of ticlopidine in the early hours following acute MI has received limited attention, perhaps be-

TABLE 6.1 — RANDOMIZED CLINICAL TRIALS OF TICLOPIDINE IN PATIENTS WITH VASCULAR DISEASE

Trial/Investigator	Study Population	Patients (n)	Treatment
Stroke and TIA			
CATS	Recent stroke	1072	Ticlopidine, 250 mg bid or placebo
TASS	Recent TIA or minor stroke	3069	Ticlopidine, 250 mg bid or ASA, 625 mg bid
TISS	Recent TIA, amaurosis fagax, or minor stroke	1632	Ticlopidine or indobufen (median doses, 250 and 200 mg bid, respectively)
PAOD			
Swedish Ticlopidine Multicentre Study	Intermittent claudication	687	Ticlopidine, 250 mg bid or placebo
Arcan, et al	Chronic intermittent claudication	169	Ticlopidine, 250 mg bid or placebo
EMATAP	Intermittent claudication	615	Ticlopidine, 250 mg bid or placebo

Unstable Angina			
Balsano, et al	Unstable angina	652	Conventional therapy with or without ticlopidine, 250 mg daily
SVG Patency			
Chevigne, et al	Coronary bypass surgery	77	Ticlopidine, 250 mg bid (started 3 days before surgery) or placebo
Limet, et al	Coronary bypass surgery	173	Ticlopidine, 250 mg bid (first dose on day 2) or placebo
Becquemin, et al	Femoropopliteal or femorofemoral bypass surgery	243	Ticlopidine, 250 mg bid or placebo
Diabetic Retinopathy			
TMD	Nonproliferative diabetic retinopathy	435	Ticlopidine, 250 mg bid or placebo

Abbreviations: ASA, aspirin; CAT, Canadian American Ticlopidine; EMATAP, Estudio Multicentrico Argentino de la Ticlopidine en las Arteriopatias Perifericas; PAOD, peripheral arterial occlusive disease; TASS, Ticlopidine Aspirin Stroke; TIA, transient ischemic attack; TISS, Ticlopidine Indobufen Stroke; TMD, Ticlopidine Microangiopathy of Diabetes; SVG, saphenous vein graft.

TABLE 6.2 — STUDY END POINTS OF RANDOMIZED CLINICAL TRIALS OF TICLOPIDINE IN PATIENTS WITH VASCULAR DISEASE

Study End Point	Follow-Up Duration	Ticlopidine Group Event Rate (%)	Comparison Group Event Rate (%)	P Value
Stroke, MI, or vascular death	Mean 2 years	11.3/y	14.8/y	0.02
Nonfatal stroke or death	3 years	17	19	0.048
Death, stroke, or MI at 1 year	—	2.9	5.8	0.004
MI, stroke, or TIA	Mean, 5.6 years	25.7	29.0	> 0.2
Cerebrovascular accident, TIA, or peripheral ischemia requiring surgery at 6 months	—	2.4	10.5	0.03
Death, MI, stroke, or cardiovascular intervention due to clinical deterioration	—	1.0	6.4	0.002
Vascular death or nonfatal MI at 6 months	—	7.3	13.6	0.009
Graft occlusion on angiography at 3 months	—	10.1	20.3	< 0.1
Graft occlusion at 360 days	—	15.9	26.1	< 0.01
Femoropopliteal or femorofemoral graft patency	2 years	82	63	0.002
Micronaneurysm progression	3 years	0.48/y	1.44/y	0.04

Abbreviations: MI, myocardial infarction; TIA, transient ischemic attack.

cause of the delayed onset (48 to 72 hours) of its antiplatelet effect. A study of patients treated with ticlopidine within 12 hours of symptom onset reported a lower peak creatine kinase concentration (suggesting reduced infarct size) compared with those not treated.[13]

■ Coronary Artery Bypass Grafting

Saphenous vein bypass conduits are prone to early occlusion that is predominantly a platelet-mediated thrombotic event. Ticlopidine (250 mg bid) has been tested against placebo beginning on postoperative day 2 in a double-blind trial of 173 patients (475 grafts). Ticlopidine significantly reduced graft occlusion on day 10 (7.1% vs 13.4%; P <0.05), day 180 (15.0% vs 24.0%; P <0.02), and day 360 (15.9% vs 26.1%; P <0.01).[14]

■ Coronary Arterial Stenting

Since its introduction by Sigwart and colleagues in 1987,[15] coronary stent implantation has been hampered by two major complications: subacute stent thrombosis and hemorrhage (related to vascular access and antithrombotic therapy regimens).

An initial report generated by the French Multicenter Registry suggested that the combination of aspirin and ticlopidine was superior to strategies that included conventional anticoagulant therapy.[16] The rates of stent thrombosis, major cardiac events, and hemorrhage were reduced with antiplatelet therapy. In a randomized study of 257 patients, the combination of ticlopidine and aspirin reduced the incidence of cardiac death, MI, repeated angioplasty, and bypass surgery (composite end point) by 75% compared with unfractionated heparin followed by warfarin (plus aspirin).[17] Subacute stent thrombosis occurred in less than 1% of patients treated with the combination antiplatelet regimen (Figure 6.1). Hemorrhagic complications occurred only in the anticoagulant therapy group. The results of several multicenter trials have confirmed these observations. Evidence provided by the Full Anticoagulation Versus Aspirin and Ticlopidine (FANTASTIC) and Multicenter Aspirin and Ticlopidine Trial After Coronary Stenting (MATTIS) trials suggest that antiplatelet strategies are superior to anticoagulant (or combined anticoagulant plus aspirin) strat-

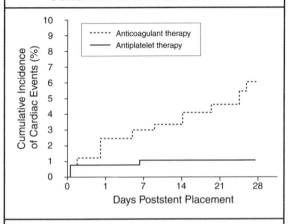

FIGURE 6.1 — REDUCED CARDIAC EVENTS WITH ANTIPLATELET THERAPY VS ANTICOAGULANT THERAPY FOLLOWING CORONARY ARTERIAL STENTING

The combination of ticlopidine and aspirin (antiplatelet therapy) reduced cardiac events by 75% following coronary arterial stenting compared with anticoagulant therapy.

Schömig A et al. *N Engl J Med.* 1996;334:1084-1089.

egies in terms of both efficacy and safety for both low- and high-risk patients.[18,19]

Although improved techniques of stent deployment, operator experience, and the development of less thrombogenic materials and design have contributed substantially to improved outcomes, the available evidence suggests that antithrombotic therapy is required for the initial 2 to 4 weeks. Whenever possible, treatment should be initiated 2 to 3 days prior to the procedure. In the EPISTENT trial,[20] ticlopidine pretreatment was associated with a significant decrease in the composite of death, MI, or target vessel revascularization at 1 year. The benefit was most robust in patients who did not receive abciximab. Some low-risk patients may only require aspirin therapy; however, combination antiplatelet therapy represents the standard of care.[21]

■ Peripheral Vascular Disease

Patients with peripheral vascular disease are known to be at risk for vascular events including:

- Stroke
- MI
- Cardiovascular death.

In a multicenter trial, 169 patients with intermittent claudication due to obstructive peripheral vascular disease were randomized in a double-blind fashion to ticlopidine (250 mg bid) or placebo.[22] At 6 months, a greater proportion of patients receiving ticlopidine had increased their walking distance and also experienced fewer cardiovascular events than those given placebo.

The Swedish Ticlopidine Multicenter Study[23] identified a nonsignificant trend favoring ticlopidine over placebo in preventing the composite clinical outcome of MI, stroke, and transient ischemic attack in patients with intermittent claudication. By "on-treatment" analysis, there was a significant benefit in favor of ticlopidine treatment.

■ Stroke

The Canadian-American Ticlopidine Study identified a clinical benefit from ticlopidine, compared with placebo, in preventing the combined primary end point of stroke, MI, or vascular disease in patients with completed stroke.[24]

The Ticlopidine Aspirin Stroke Study[25] was designed to determine the comparative benefits of ticlopidine (250 mg bid) over aspirin (1300 mg/d) in 3069 patients with recent transient or mild persistent focal cerebral or retinal ischemia. The 3-year event rate for nonfatal stroke or death (from any cause) was 17% for ticlopidine-treated and 19% for aspirin-treated patients (12% reduction; $P = 0.048$). The rates of fatal and nonfatal stroke at 3 years were 10% and 13%, respectively (21% risk reduction; $P = 0.024$).

The comparative benefit of ticlopidine (or clopidogrel) vs dipyridamole/aspirin combination therapy (Aggrenox) is currently unknown.

Summary

Ticlopidine is a thienopyridine derivative that inhibits ADP-mediated platelet aggregation. Because of its requirement for hepatic metabolism to an active compound, the platelet-inhibiting properties of ticlopidine (when given in currently recommended doses) are delayed for 2 to 3 days after treatment initiation. The available evidence suggests that ticlopidine offers benefit following coronary stenting, where in combination with aspirin, subacute stent thrombosis is reduced. Ticlopidine can also be used in patients with coronary artery disease who are unable to take aspirin (because of true allergy or an adverse reaction). Bone marrow suppression and TTP are ticlopidine's side effects that cause the most concern and therefore careful monitoring is recommended when treatment is continued beyond 14 days. The more favorable safety profile of clopidogrel coupled with its proven benefit in a wide variety of patients with atherosclerotic vascular disease supports preferential use.

REFERENCES

1. Bruno JJ. The mechanism of action of ticlopidine. *Thromb Res.* 1983;4(suppl):59-67.

2. Piovella F, Ricetti MM, Almasioni P, Samaden A, Semino G, Ascari E. The effect of ticlopidine on human endothelial cells in culture. *Thromb Res.* 1984;33:323-332.

3. O'Brien JR, Etherington MD, Shuttleworth RD. Ticlopidine—an antiplatelet drug: effects in human volunteers. *Thromb Res.* 1978;13:245-254.

4. Ellis DJ, Roe RL, Bruno JJ, et al. The effects of ticlopidine hydrochloride on bleeding and platelet function in man. *Thromb Haemost.* 1981;46:176. Abstract.

5. De Caterina R, Sicari R, Bernini W, Lazzerini G, Buti Strata G, Giannessi D. Benefit/risk profile of combined antiplatelet therapy with ticlopidine and aspirin. *Thromb Haemost.* 1991;65:504-510.

6. De Minno G, Cerbone AM, Mattioli PL, Turco S, Iovine C, Mancini M. Functionally thromboasthenic state in normal platelets following the administration of ticlopidine. *J Clin Invest.* 1985;75:328-338.

7. Panak E, Blanchard J, Roe RL. Evaluation of the antithrombotic efficacy of ticlopidine in man. *Agents Actions Suppl*. 1984;15:148-166.

8. Bennett CL, Weinberg PD, Rozenberg-Ben-Dror K, Yarnold PR, Kwaan HC, Green D. Thrombotic thrombocytopenic purpura associated with ticlopidine. A review of 60 cases. *Ann Intern Med*. 1998;128:541-544.

9. Steinhubl SR, Tan WA, Foody JM, Topol EJ for the EPISTENT Investigators. Incidence and clinical course of thrombotic thrombocytopenic purpura due to ticlopidine following coronary stenting. *JAMA*. 1999;281:806-810.

10. Berglund U, von Schenck H, Wallentin L. Effects of ticlopidine on platelet function in men with stable angina pectoris. *Thromb Haemost*. 1985;54:808-812.

11. Berglund U, Lassvik C, Wallentin L. Effects of the platelet inhibitor ticlopidine on exercise tolerance in stable angina pectoris. *Eur Heart J*. 1987;8:25-30.

12. Balsano F, Rizzon P, Violi F, et al. Antiplatelet treatment with ticlopidine in unstable angina. A controlled multicenter clinical trial. The Studio della Ticlopidina nell'Angina Instabile Group. *Circulation*. 1990;82:17-26.

13. Knudsen JB, Kjoller E, Skagen K, Gormsen J. The effect of ticlopidine on platelet functions in acute myocardial infarction. A double blind controlled trial. *Thromb Haemost*. 1985;53:332-336.

14. Limet R, David JL, Magotteaux P, Larock MP, Rigo P. Prevention of aorta-coronary bypass graft occlusion. Beneficial effect of ticlopidine on early and late patency rates of venous coronary bypass grafts: a double-blind study. *J Thorac Cardiovasc Surg*. 1987;94:773-783.

15. Sigwart U, Puel J, Mirkovitch V, Joffre F, Kappenberger L. Intravascular stents to prevent occlusion and restenosis after transluminal angioplasty. *N Engl J Med*. 1987;316:701-706.

16. Morice MC, Zemour G, Benveniste E, et al. Intracoronary stenting without coumadin: one month results of a French multicenter study. *Cathet Cardiovasc Diagn*. 1995;35:1-7.

17. Schömig A, Neumann FJ, Kastrati A, et al. A randomized comparison of antiplatelet and anticoagulant therapy after the placement of coronary-artery stents. *N Engl J Med*. 1996;334:1084-1089.

18. Bertrand ME, Legrand V, Boland J, et al. Randomized multicenter comparison of conventional anticoagulation versus antiplatelet therapy in unplanned and elective coronary stenting. The Full Anticoagulation Versus Aspirin and Ticlopidine (FANTASTIC) Study. *Circulation*. 1998;98:1597-1603.

19. Urban P, Macaya C, Rupprecht HJ, et al for the MATTIS Investigators. Randomized evaluation of anticoagulation versus antiplatelet therapy after coronary stent implantation in high risk patients: the Multicenter Aspirin and Ticlopidine Trial After Intracoronary Stenting (MATTIS). *Circulation*. 1998;98:2126-2132.

20. Steinhubl SR, Ellis SG, Wolski K, Lincoff AM, Topol EJ, for the EPISTENT Investigators Ticlopidine pretreatment before coronary stenting is associated with sustained decrease in adverse cardiac events. *Circulation*. 2001;103:1403-1409.

21. Leon MB, Baim DS, Gordon P, et al. Clinical and angiographic results from the stent anticoagulation regimen study (STARS). *Circulation*. 1996:94(suppl I):I-685.

22. Arcan JC, Blanchard J, Boissel JP, Destors JM, Panak E. Multicenter double-blind study of ticlopidine in the treatment of intermittent claudication and the prevention of its complications. *Angiology*. 1988;39:802-811.

23. Janzon L, Bergqvist D, Boberg J, et al. Prevention of myocardial infarction and stroke in patients with intermittent claudication: effects of ticlopidine. Results from STIMS, the Swedish Ticlopidine Multicenter Study. *J Intern Med*. 1990;227:301-308.

24. Gent M, Blakely JA, Easton JD, et al. The Canadian-American Ticlopidine Study (CATS) in thromboembolic stroke. *Lancet*. 1989;1:1215-1220.

25. Hass WK, Easton JD, Adams HP, et al. A randomized trial comparing ticlopidine hydrochloride with aspirin for the prevention of stroke in high risk patients. Ticlopidine Aspirin Stroke Study Group. *N Engl J Med*. 1989;321:501-507.

7   Clopidogrel

Clopidogrel is a novel platelet antagonist that is several times more potent than ticlopidine, but associated with fewer adverse effects.

In Vitro and Ex Vivo Effect on Platelets

After repeated 75-mg oral doses of clopidogrel, plasma concentrations of the parent compound, which has no platelet inhibiting effect, are very low. Clopidogrel is extensively metabolized in the liver. The main circulating metabolite is a carboxylic acid derivative with a plasma elimination half-life of 7.7 ± 2.3 hours. Approximately 50% of an oral dose is excreted in the urine and the remaining 50% in feces over the following 5 days.

Dose-dependent inhibition of platelet aggregation is observed 2 hours after a single oral dose of clopidogrel with significant inhibition achieved with loading doses (≥ 300 mg) (Figure 7.1). Repeated doses of 75-mg clopidogrel per day inhibit adenosine diphosphate (ADP)-mediated aggregation on the first day and inhibition reaches steady state between day 3 and day 7. At steady state, the average inhibition of ADP is between 40% and 60%.

Based on *ex vivo* studies, clopidogrel is approximately 100-fold more potent than ticlopidine. There are no cumulative antiplatelet effects with prolonged oral administration.

The combined administration of clopidogrel (300-mg loading dose) and aspirin yields a readily discernible antithrombotic effect within 90 to 120 minutes.[1,2]

Mechanism of Action

Clopidogrel selectively inhibits the binding of ADP to its platelet receptor (P2Y$_{12}$) and the subsequent G-protein linked mobilization of intracellular calcium and activation of the glycoprotein (GP)IIb/IIIa complex.[3,4] The specific re-

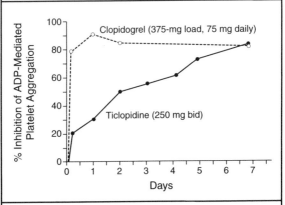

**FIGURE 7.1 — INHIBITION OF
ADP-MEDIATED PLATELET AGGREGATION
WITH CLOPIDOGREL VS TICLOPIDINE**

Clopidogrel (375-mg load, 75 mg daily)

Ticlopidine (250 mg bid)

% Inhibition of ADP-Mediated Platelet Aggregation

Days

Inhibited adenosine diphosphate (ADP)-mediated platelet aggregation as a function of time with a "front-loaded" clopidogrel dosing strategy vs ticlopidine.

ceptor has been cloned and is abundantly present on the platelet surface.[5,6] Clopidogrel has no direct effect on cyclooxygenase, phosphodiesterase, or adenosine uptake.

Absorption

Clopidogrel is rapidly absorbed following oral administration with peak plasma levels of the predominant circulating metabolite occurring 1 hour later. Administration with meals does not significantly modify the bioavailability of clopidogrel. No dose adjustment is required for elderly patients, women, or those with renal impairment.

Safety

The available information suggests that clopidogrel offers safety advantages over ticlopidine, particularly with regard to bone marrow suppression and other hematologic abnormalities. Although thrombotic thrombocytopenic purpura (TTP) has been reported with clopidogrel,[7] its occurrence (11 cases per 3 million patients treated) is rare, and has not been reported in clinical trials performed to date.

Clinical Experience

■ Vascular Disease

The well-documented benefit derived from platelet inhibition in patients with vascular disease, coupled with a concerning adverse-effect profile witnessed with aspirin and ticlopidine, fostered the rapid development of clopidogrel as a potential alternative to existing therapies. The Clopidogrel versus Aspirin in Patients at Risk for Ischemic Events (CAPRIE) Study[8] was designed to test the hypothesis that clopidogrel (75 mg daily) would reduce vascular events in high-risk patients by approximately 15% compared with aspirin (325 mg daily). The study population consisted of patients with atherosclerotic vascular disease manifested as recent ischemic stroke, recent myocardial infarction (MI), or symptomatic peripheral arterial occlusive disease. A total of 19,185 patients were enrolled in the international trial. The mean follow-up was 1.91 years. Patients treated with clopidogrel (by intention-to-treat analysis) had a 5.32% annual risk of ischemic stroke, MI, or vascular death compared with 5.83% among aspirin-treated patients (Table 7.1, Figure 7.2) (relative risk reduction 8.7%; 95% confidence interval [CI] 0.3 to 16.5; $P = 0.043$). A corresponding "on-treatment" analysis yielded a relative risk reduction of 9.4%.

Although CAPRIE was not powered to identify differences in specific subsets, for patients experiencing a stroke, the average event rate per year in the clopidogrel group was 7.15% compared with 7.71% in the aspirin group (relative-reduction 7.3%; $P = 0.26$). For patients with MI, the average event rate per year was 5.03% in the clopidogrel group compared with 4.84% in the aspirin group (relative risk increase 3.7%; $P = 0.66$). In contrast, patients with peripheral vascular disease experienced a 3.71% annual event rate with clopidogrel and a 4.86% rate with aspirin (relative-risk reduction 23.8%; $P = 0.002$).

Although there were no major differences in safety between treatment groups, a greater proportion of patients re-

Outcome Event Cluster and Treatment Group	First Outcome Events			Event Rate (%/y)	Relative-Risk ↓ (95% CI)	P Value
	Nonfatal	Fatal	Total			
Ischemic stroke, MI, or vascular death (primary cluster)						
Clopidogrel (nyrs = 17,636*)	631	308	939	5.32	8.7% (0.3-16.5)	0.043
Aspirin (nyrs = 17,519)	700	321	1021	5.83		
Ischemic stroke, MI, or vascular death						
Clopidogrel (nyrs = 17,594)	677	302	979	5.56	7.6% (−0.8-15.3)	0.076
Aspirin (nyrs = 17,482)	737	314	1051	6.01		
Vascular death						
Clopidogrel (nyrs = 17,482)	—	350	350	1.90	7.6% (6.9-20.1)	0.29
Aspirin (nyrs = 18,354)	—	378	378	2.06		

TABLE 7.1 — CLINICAL OUTCOMES IN CAPRIE (INTENTION-TO-TREAT ANALYSIS)

					Relative-risk reduction (95% CI)	P value
Any† stroke, MI, or death from any cause						
Clopidogrel (nyrs = 17,622)	643	490	1133	6.43	7.0% (–0.9-14.2)	0.081
Aspirin (nyrs = 17,501)	720	487	1207	6.90		
Death from any cause						
Clopidogrel (nyrs = 18,377)	–	560	560	3.05	2.2% (–9.9-12.9)	0.71
Aspirin (nyrs = 18,354)	–	571	571	3.11		

Abbreviations: CI, confidence interval; MI, myocardial infarction.

* Patient-years at risk for outcome cluster.
† Includes primary intracranial hemorrhage.

From: CAPRIE Steering Committee. *Lancet.* 1996;348:1329-1339.

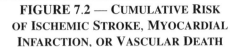

FIGURE 7.2 — CUMULATIVE RISK OF ISCHEMIC STROKE, MYOCARDIAL INFARCTION, OR VASCULAR DEATH

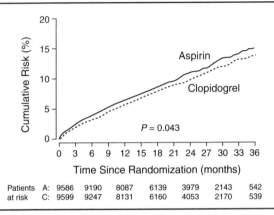

Cumulative risk of ischemic stroke, myocardial infarction, or vascular death in the CAPRIE Study. Event rates were lower with clopidogrel than aspirin.

CAPRIE Steering Committee. *Lancet*. 1996;348:1329-1339.

ceiving aspirin had the study drug permanently discontinued because of gastrointestinal hemorrhage, indigestion, nausea, or vomiting. Approximately one out of every 1000 patients treated with clopidogrel experienced neutropenia ($<1.2 \times 10^9$/L) (similar to aspirin treatment); however, cases of TTP were not reported.

In the CAPRIE study,[9] all-cause mortality, vascular death, MI, stroke, and rehospitalization were determined for 1480 patients who had previously undergone bypass grafting. Those randomized to clopidogrel had a 31.2% relative risk reduction of events compared with aspirin treatment (Figure 7.3). Considering the composite end point used in the main CAPRIE trial—vascular death, MI, or ischemic stroke—a 36.3% relative reduction was seen with clopidogrel (5.8% per year) compared with aspirin (9.1% per year) ($P = 0.004$).

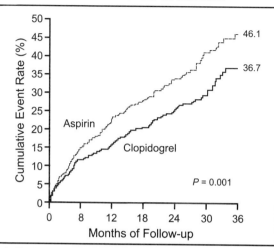

■ **Coronary Stenting**

A multicenter, randomized, controlled trial, Clopidogrel Plus ASA vs Ticlodipine Plus ASA in Stent Patients Study (CLASSICS)[10] included 1020 patients undergoing coronary stent placement who received either aspirin (325 mg qd) plus ticlopidine (250 mg bid), aspirin plus clopidogrel (75 mg daily), or aspirin plus front-loaded clopidogrel (300 mg as an initial dose followed by 75 mg qd). Treatment was continued for 28 days after stent placement. Intravenous GPIIb/IIIa antagonists were not administered to patients enrolled in the trial. The primary safety end point was a composite of neutropenia, thrombocytopenia, bleeding, and drug discontinuation for adverse events (noncardiac). The secondary efficacy end point was a composite of MI, target vessel revascularization, and cardiovascular death.

The primary end point was experienced by 9.1% of ticlopidine-treated patients, 6.3% of clopidogrel-treated patients (75 mg), and 2.9% of front-loaded clopidogrel-treated patients. Early drug discontinuation occurred in 8.2%, 5.1%, and 2.0% of patients, respectively. The most commonly reported adverse effects prompting drug discontinuation were allergic reactions, gastrointestinal distress, and skin rashes. The secondary cardiovascular end points were reached by 0.9%, 1.5%, and 1.3% of patients, respectively.

In patients undergoing coronary arterial stent placement, clopidogrel (plus aspirin) compares favorably with ticlopidine in preventing thrombotic closure; however, it is associated with fewer noncardiac adverse events that cause discontinuation of treatment.[11]

The importance of adequate platelet inhibition both preceding and following PCI (with stenting) was confirmed in the PCI-CURE study.[12] A total of 2658 patients undergoing PCI were randomized to double-blind treatment with clopidogrel or placebo (aspirin alone) for, on average, 6 days before the procedure followed by 4 weeks of open-label thienopyridine (after which study drug was resumed for 8 months). The primary end point (cardiovascular death, MI, or urgent target vessel revascularization within 30 days) was reached in 4.5% of clopidogrel-treated patients and 6.4% of placebo-treated patients (30% relative reduction) (Figure 7.4). Long-term administration of clopidogrel was associated with a lower rate of death, MI, or any revascularization with no increased bleeding complications (Figure 7.5).

The TARGET trial[13] investigated the safety and efficiency of two GPIIb/IIIa receptor antagonists in patients undergoing PCI (with the intent to perform stenting). All patients received aspirin and when possible, clopidogrel (300 mg) 2 to 6 hours before the procedure. Both antiplatelet agents were continued throughout the study period. Urgent target vessel revascularization (<1.0%) and MI (CK >5 times normal) were low in both groups, as was major hemorrhage.

Intracoronary radiation therapy is an available means to treat in-stent restenosis; however, late total occlusion and thrombosis are serious complications with rates approaching 10% to 15%. Accumulating evidence suggests that pro-

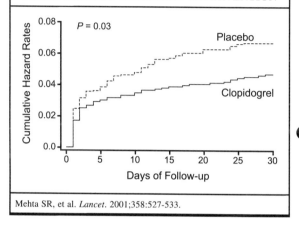

FIGURE 7.4 — KAPLAN-MEIER CUMULATIVE HAZARD RATES FOR PRIMARY OUTCOME OF CARDIOVASCULAR DEATH, MYOCARDIAL INFARCTION, OR URGENT TARGET-VESSEL REVASCULARIZATION AT 30 DAYS AFTER PERCUTANEOUS CORONARY INTERVENTION

Mehta SR, et al. *Lancet.* 2001;358:527-533.

longed treatment with clopidogrel and aspirin (6 months or more) is a more effective means to prevent late thrombosis than an abbreviated course (1 month).[14]

■ **Acute Coronary Syndromes**

The benefit of continued therapy with aspirin and clopidogrel was confirmed in the Clopidogrel in Unstable Angina to Prevent Recurrent Events (CURE) trial.[15] A total of 12,562 patients experiencing an acute coronary syndrome without ST-segment elevation received clopidogrel (300 mg immediately, 75 mg daily) plus aspirin (75 to 325 mg daily) or aspirin alone for 3 to 12 months. The composite of death, MI, or stroke occurred in 9.3% and 11.4% of patients, respectively (relative risk reduction 20%). In hospital refractory ischemia, congestive heart failure and revascularization procedures were also less likely in clopidogrel-treated patients (Figures 7.6 and 7.7). Although there was a greater risk of major hemorrhage with combi-

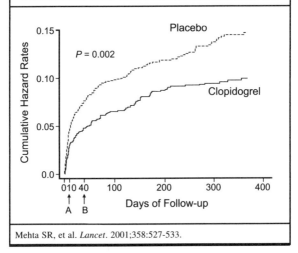

FIGURE 7.5 — KAPLAN-MEIER CUMULATIVE HAZARD RATES FOR CARDIOVASCULAR DEATH OR MYOCARDIAL INFARCTION FROM RANDOMIZATION TO FOLLOW-UP AFTER PERCUTANEOUS CORONARY INTERVENTION

Placebo

$P = 0.002$

Clopidogrel

Mehta SR, et al. *Lancet*. 2001;358:527-533.

nation therapy, life-threatening bleeding and hemorrhagic strokes occurred with similar frequency between groups.

Summary

Clopidogrel (Plavix) is an effective inhibitor of ADP-mediated platelet aggregation. Like ticlopidine, clopidogrel must first be hepatically transformed to its active metabolite to exhibit platelet-inhibiting properties. With mounting clinical trial-based and clinical experience, clopidogrel appears to offer benefit in patients with atherothrombosis of the cardiovascular, peripheral vascular, and cerebrovascular systems where its administration reduces cardiac events to a greater degree than aspirin. Clopidogrel in combination with aspirin also represents the current standard of care following coronary stent placement and in patients with acute coronary syndromes.

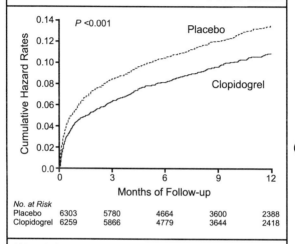

FIGURE 7.6 — CUMULATIVE HAZARD RATES FOR THE FIRST PRIMARY OUTCOME OF DEATH FROM CARDIOVASCULAR CAUSES, NONFATAL MYOCARDIAL INFARCTION, OR STROKE DURING THE 12 MONTHS OF THE CURE TRIAL

No. at Risk					
Placebo	6303	5780	4664	3600	2388
Clopidogrel	6259	5866	4779	3644	2418

Abbreviation: CURE [trial], Clopidogrel in Unstable Angina to Prevent Recurrent Events.

The Clopidogrel in Unstable Angina to Prevent Recurrent Events Trial Investigators. *N Engl J Med*. 2001;345:494-502.

REFERENCES

1. Cadroy Y, Bossavy JP, Thalamas C, Sagnard L, Sakariassen K, Boneu B. Early potent antithrombotic effect with combined aspirin and a loading dose of clopidogrel on experimental arterial thrombogenesis in humans. *Circulation*. 2000;101:2823-2828.

2. Helft G, Osende JI, Worthley SG, et al. Acute antithrombotic effect of a front loaded regimen of clopidogrel in patients with atherosclerosis on aspirin. *Arterioscler Thromb Vasc Biol*. 2000;20:2316-2321.

3. Gachet C, Stierlé A, Cazenave JP, et al. The thienopyridine PCR 4099 selectively inhibits ADP-induced platelet aggregation and fibrinogen binding without modifying the membrane glycoprotein IIb-IIIa complex in rat and in man. *Biochem Pharmacol*. 1990;40:229-238.

FIGURE 7.7 — RATES AND RELATIVE RISKS OF THE FIRST PRIMARY OUTCOME OF DEATH FROM CARDIOVASCULAR CAUSES, NONFATAL MYOCARDIAL INFARCTION, OR STROKE IN VARIOUS SUBGROUPS WITH CONSISTENCY OF BENEFIT WITH CLOPIDOGREL

Characteristic	No. of Patients	Patients With Event (%)	
		Placebo	Clopidogrel
Overall	12562	11.4	9.3
Associated myocardial infarction	3283	13.7	11.3
No associated myocardial infarction	9279	10.6	8.6
Male sex	7726	11.9	9.1
Female sex	4836	10.7	9.5
<65 yr old	6354	7.6	5.4
>65 yr old	6208	15.3	13.3
ST-segment deviation	6275	14.3	11.5
No ST-segment deviation	6287	8.6	7.0
Enzymes elevated at entry	3176	13.0	10.7
Enzymes not elevated at entry	9386	10.9	8.8

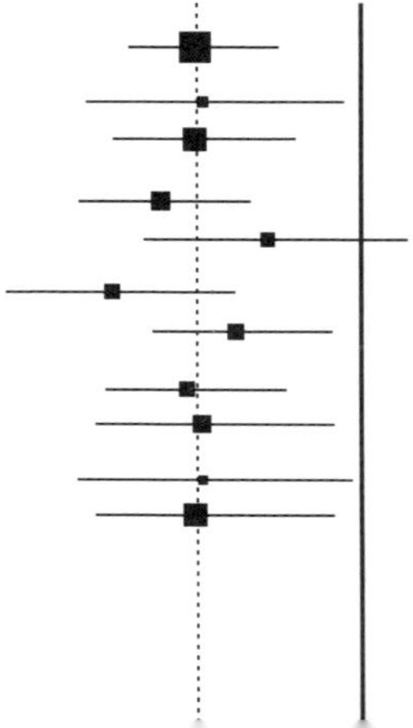

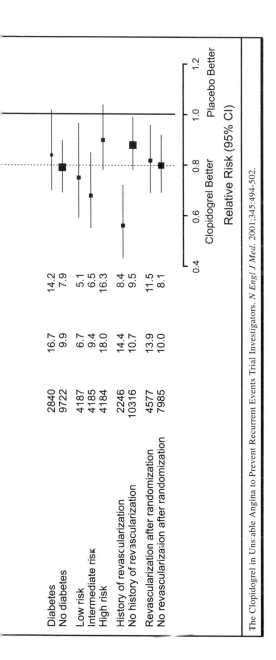

Diabetes	2840	16.7	14.2
No diabetes	9722	9.9	7.9
Low risk	4187	6.7	5.1
Intermediate risk	4185	9.4	6.5
High risk	4184	18.0	16.3
History of revascularization	2246	14.4	8.4
No history of revascularization	10316	10.7	9.5
Revascularization after randomization	4577	13.9	11.5
No revascularization after randomization	7985	10.0	8.1

Relative Risk (95% CI)

Clopidogrel Better   Placebo Better

0.4   0.6   0.8   1.0   1.2

4. Gachet C, Savi P, Ohlmann P, Maffrand JP, Jakobs KH, Cazenave JP. ADP receptor induced activation of guanine nucleotide binding proteins in rat platelet membranes—an effect selectively blocked by the thienopyridine clopidogrel. *Thromb Haemost.* 1992;68:79-83.

5. Mills DC, Puri R, Hu CJ, et al. Clopidogrel inhibits the binding of ADP analogues to the receptor mediating inhibition of platelet adenylate cyclase. *Arterioscler Thromb.* 1992;12:430-436.

6. Hollopeter G, Jantzen HM, Vincent D, et al. Identification of the platelet ADP receptor targeted by antithrombotic drugs. *Nature.* 2001;409:202-207.

7. Bennett CL, Connors JM, Carwile JM, et al. Thrombotic thrombocytopenia purpura associated with clopidogrel. *N Engl J Med.* 2000;342:1773-1777.

8. CAPRIE Steering Committee. A randomised, blinded, trial of clopidogrel versus aspirin in patients at risk of ischaemic events (CAPRIE). *Lancet.* 1996;348:1329-1339.

9. Bhatt DL, Chew DP, Hirsch AT, Ringleb PA, Hacke W, Topol EJ. Superiority of clopidogrel versus aspirin in patients with prior cardiac surgery. *Circulation.* 2001;103:363-368.

10. Bertrand ME. Double-blind study of the safety of clopidogrel with and without a loading dose in combination with aspirin compared with ticlopidine in combination with aspirin after coronary stenting: the Clopidogrel Aspirin Stent International Cooperative Study (CLASSICS). *Circulation.* 2000;102:624-629.

11. Muller C, Buttner HJ, Peterson J, Roskamm H. A randomized comparison of clopidogrel and aspirin versus ticlopidine and aspirin after the placement of coronary-artery stents. *Circulation.* 2000;101: 590-593.

12. Mehta SR, Yusuf S, Peters RJ, for the CURE Investigators. Effects of pretreatment with clopidogrel and aspirin followed by long-term therapy in patients undergoing percutaneous coronary intervention: the PCI-CURE Study. *Lancet.* 2001;358:527-533.

13. Topol EJ, Moliterno DJ, Herrman HC, et al. Comparison of two platelet glycoprotein IIb/IIIa inhibitors, tirofiban and abciximab, for the prevention of ischemic events with percutaneous coronary revascularization. *N Engl J Med.* 2001;344:1888-1894.

14. Waksman R, Ajani AE, White RL, et al. Prolonged antiplatelet therapy to prevent late thrombosis after intracoronary γ-radiation in patients with restenosis: Washington Radiation for In-Stent Restenosis Trial plus 6 months of clopidogrel (WRIST PLUS). *Circulation.* 2001;103:2332-2335.

15. The Clopidogrel in Unstable Angina to Prevent Recurrent Events Trial Investigators. Effects of clopidogrel in addition to aspirin in patients with acute coronary syndromes without ST-segment elevation. *N Engl J Med.* 2001;345:494-502.

7

8
Platelet Glycoprotein IIb/IIIa Receptor Antagonists

The glycoprotein (GP) IIb/IIIa (αIIb/β_3) receptor represents a final common pathway for platelet aggregation in response to a wide variety of biochemical and mechanical agonists. Accordingly, it represents an attractive target for therapies that can be applied to patients with acute coronary syndromes in whom platelet activation is heightened substantially and represents the predominant pathobiologic substrate.

Intravenous Platelet GPIIb/IIIa Receptor Antagonists

8

The evolution of GPIIb/IIIa receptor antagonists represents a true "bench-to-bedside" metamorphosis that began with murine monoclonal antibodies and more recently has focused on small peptide or nonpeptide molecules that have structural similarities to fibrinogen and other circulating ligands. There are three intravenous GPIIb/IIIa receptor antagonists that have been approved by the Food and Drug Administration:

- Abciximab (ReoPro)
- Tirofiban (Aggrastat)
- Eptifibatide (Integrilin).

■ Abciximab

Abciximab (ReoPro) is the Fab fragment of the chimeric human-murine monoclonal antibody c7E3.

Pharmacokinetics

Following an intravenous bolus, free plasma concentrations of abciximab decrease rapidly with an initial half-life of less than 10 minutes and a second-phase half-life of 30 minutes, representing rapid binding to the platelet GPIIb/IIIa receptor. Abciximab remains in the circulation for 10 or more days in the platelet-bound state.

Pharmacodynamics

Intravenous administration of abciximab in doses ranging from 0.15 mg/kg to 0.3 mg/kg produces a rapid dose-dependent inhibition of platelet aggregation in response to adenosine diphosphate (ADP). At the highest dose, 80% of platelet GPIIb/IIIa receptors are occupied within 2 hours and platelet aggregation, even with 20mM ADP, is completely inhibited. Sustained inhibition is achieved with prolonged infusions (12 to 24 hours) and low-level receptor blockade is present for up to 10 days following cessation of the infusion; however, platelet inhibition during infusions beyond 24 hours has not been well characterized. Platelet aggregation in response to 5 mM ADP returns to ≥50% of baseline within 24 hours in a majority of cases (Figure 8.1).

Clinical Experience

In nearly 2100 patients undergoing either balloon coronary angioplasty or atherectomy who were judged to be at high risk for ischemic (thrombotic) complications, a bolus of abciximab (0.25 mg/kg) followed by a 12-hour continuous infusion (10 μg/min) was found to reduce the occurrence of death, myocardial infarction (MI), or the need for an urgent intervention (repeat angioplasty, stent placement, balloon pump insertion, or bypass grafting) by 35%.[1] At 6 months,[2] the absolute difference in patients with a major ischemic event or elective revascularization was 8.1% comparing patients who received abciximab (bolus plus infusion) with those given placebo (35.1% vs 27.0%; 23% reduction). All patients received aspirin and unfractionated heparin during the procedure. At 3 years,[3] the composite end point occurred in:

- 41.1% of those receiving an abciximab bolus plus infusion
- 47.4% of those receiving an abciximab bolus only
- 47.2% of those receiving placebo.

The greatest benefit was observed in patients with refractory angina or evolving MI (Table 8.1).

The Evaluation in PTCA to Improve Long-term Outcome with Abciximab GPIIb/IIIa Blockade (EPILOG) study[4] included 2792 patients undergoing elective or urgent percutaneous coronary revascularization who received ei-

FIGURE 8.1 — DURATION OF GPIIb/IIIa RECEPTOR BLOCKADE AND INHIBITION OF PLATELET AGGREGATION WITH ABCIXIMAB

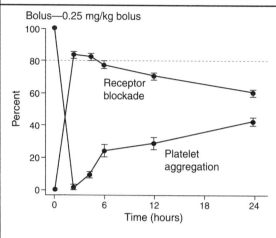

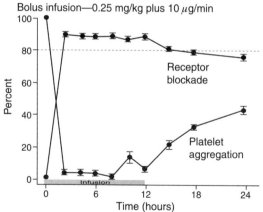

Duration of receptor blockade and inhibition of platelet aggregation (5 μM ADP) (*top*) in 5 patients receiving a 0.25 mg/kg bolus dose of abciximab and (*bottom*) in 5 patients receiving a 0.25 mg/kg bolus plus a 24-h infusion of 10 μg/min. Data are presented as the mean ± SEM.

Uprichard A. *Handbook of Experimental Pharmacology*. Berlin, Germany: Springer-Verlag. 1999;175-208,

End Point	Placebo (n = 696)	Bolus (n = 698)	Bolus + Infusion (n = 708)	P Value*	Odds Ratio (95% CI)*
Composite					
1 year	266 (38.6)	251 (36.3)	216 (30.8)	.002	0.75 (0.63-0.90)
2 years	290 (42.3)	290 (42.4)	253 (36.3)	.009	0.80 (0.68-0.95)
3 years	319 (47.2)	321 (47.4)	283 (41.1)	.009	0.81 (0.69-0.95)
Death					
1 year	31 (4.5)	29 (4.2)	30 (4.2)	.841	0.95 (0.58-1.57)
2 years	46 (6.6)	40 (5.8)	37 (5.2)	.277	0.79 (0.51-1.22)
3 years	59 (8.6)	54 (8.0)	47 (6.8)	.202	0.78 (0.53-1.14)

TABLE 8.1 — CLINICAL TRIALS OF ABCIXIMAB (REOPRO): LONG-TERM FOLLOW-UP IN THE EPIC STUDY

				P value	Odds ratio (95% CI)
Myocardial infarction					
1 year	77 (11.2)	62 (9.0)	55 (7.9)	.032	0.69 (0.49-0.97)
2 years	84 (12.4)	73 (10.8)	64 (9.3)	.057	0.73 (0.53-1.01)
3 years	91 (13.6)	81 (12.2)	72 (10.7)	.075	0.76 (0.56-1.03)
Revascularization					
1 year	221 (32.6)	207 (30.4)	178 (25.6)	.004	0.75 (0.62-0.91)
2 years	242 (36.0)	237 (35.3)	207 (30.2)	.013	0.79 (0.66-0.95)
3 years	265 (40.1)	256 (38.6)	234 (34.8)	.021	0.81 (0.68-0.97)

Abbreviations: CI, confidence interval; EPIC, Evaluation of Platelet IIb/IIIa Inhibition for Prevention of Ischemic Complications [study].

* *P* values and odds ratio represent the comparison of bolus + infusion vs placebo. All values are No. (%) except where otherwise indicated.

From: Topol EJ, et al. *JAMA*. 1997;278:479-484.

8

ther abciximab with standard, weight-adjusted unfractionated heparin (initial bolus 100 U/kg, target activated clotting time [ACT] $\geq$300 seconds); abciximab with low-dose, weight-adjusted heparin (initial bolus 70 U/kg, target ACT 200 seconds); or placebo with standard-dose, weight-adjusted heparin. At 30 days, the composite event rate was 5.4%, 5.2%, and 11.7%, respectively. The benefit was observed in both high-risk and low-risk patients.

The c7E3 Fab Antiplatelet Therapy in Unstable Refractory Angina (CAPTURE) study[5] was uniquely designed to assess whether abciximab, given during the 18 to 24 hours before coronary angioplasty, could improve outcome in patients with refractory (myocardial ischemia despite nitrates, heparin, and aspirin) unstable angina. A total of 1265 patients (of 1400 scheduled) were randomly assigned to abciximab or placebo. By 30 days, the primary end point (death, MI, urgent revascularization) occurred in 11.3% of abciximab-treated patients and in 15.9% of placebo-treated patients ($P = 0.012$). The rate of MI was lower *before* and *during* coronary interventions in those given abciximab.

Patients participating in the Global Use of Strategies to Open Occluded Arteries (GUSTO) IV-ACS trial[6] had chest pain and either ST-segment depression or elevated troponin levels. They were randomized to receive placebo, abciximab for 24 hours, or abciximab for 48 hours with recommended avoidance of revascularization during the initial 48 hours. Neither abciximab group fared better than placebo with respect to death or MI at 30 days. The overall event rates were low.

The Abciximab Before Direct Angioplasty and Stenting in Myocardial Infarction Regarding Acute and Long-Term Follow-up (ADMIRAL) trial[7] included 300 patients with acute ST-segment elevation MI who underwent percutaneous coronary intervention (PCI) (plus stenting) and received either abciximab or placebo. At 30 days, a composite of death, reinfarction, or urgent revascularization (target vessel) had occurred in 6% of abciximab-treated and 14.6% of placebo-treated patients; at 6 months, the corresponding figures were 7.4% and 15.9%, respectively. The early administration of abciximab improved coronary patency before stenting, the success rate of the procedures, and the rate of patency 6 months after the procedure.

Arterial thrombi are composed of platelets and fibrin. Accordingly, the combined administration of GPIIb/IIIa receptor antagonists and fibrinolytics makes sound biologic sense and has been shown to improve both epicardial and microvascular coronary blood flow in the setting of acute MI (Figure 8.2).[8]

In the GUSTO V study,[9] 16,588 patients with acute ST-segment elevation MI received either reteplase (standard dose) or half-dose reteplase plus abciximab. Although the 30-day mortality rates did not differ significantly, there were fewer deaths or reinfarctions with combined therapy. Similarly, there was less need for urgent revascularization and fewer nonfatal ischemic complications of MI with reteplase plus abciximab compared with reteplase alone. Intracranial hemorrhage rates did not differ between treatments; however, moderate-to-severe bleeding was more likely with

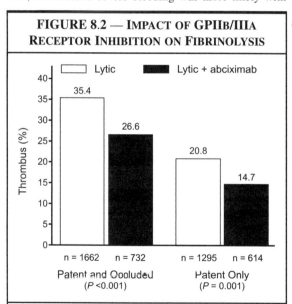

FIGURE 8.2 — IMPACT OF GPIIb/IIIa RECEPTOR INHIBITION ON FIBRINOLYSIS

Angiographically evident thrombus was reduced with the combined administration of a fibrinolytic (predominately tissue plasminogen activator [tPA]) and abciximab.

Gibson CM, et al. *Circulation.* 2001;103:2550-2554.

combined therapy and patients >75 years of age were at increased risk for hemorrhagic stroke (odds ratio 1.91). All patients in GUSTO V received unfractionated heparin and aspirin.

■ Tirofiban

Tirofiban (Aggrastat), a tyrosine derivative with a molecular weight of 495 kd, is a nonpeptide inhibitor (peptidomimetic) of the platelet GPIIb/IIIa receptor.

Pharmacodynamics

Tirofiban, like other nonpeptides, mimics the geometric, stereotactic, and change characteristics of the RGD sequence, thus interfering with platelet aggregation.

Three doses of tirofiban were studied in a phase I study of patients undergoing coronary angioplasty who received one of three graduated regimens intravenously with a bolus dose of 5, 10 or 15 μg/kg and a continuous (16- to 24-hour) infusion of 0.05, 0.10, or 0.15 μg/kg/min.[10] A dose-dependent inhibition of *ex vivo* platelet aggregation was observed within minutes of bolus administration and was sustained during the continuous infusion.

Clinical Trials and Experience

The Randomized Efficacy Study of Tirofiban Outcomes and Restenosis (RESTORE) trial[11] was a randomized, double-blind, placebo-controlled trial of tirofiban in patients undergoing coronary intervention within 72 hours of hospital presentation with an acute coronary syndrome.

Patients (n = 2139) received tirofiban as a 10 μg/kg intravenous bolus over a 3-minute period and a continuous infusion of 0.15 μg/kg/min over 36 hours. All patients received heparin and aspirin. The primary composite end point (death, MI, angioplasty failure requiring bypass surgery or unplanned stent placement, recurrent ischemia requiring repeat angioplasty) at 30 days was reduced from 12.2% in the placebo group to 10.3% in the tirofiban group (16% relative reduction).

The Platelet Receptor Inhibition in Ischemic Syndrome Management (PRISM) trial[12] included 3231 patients with unstable angina/non–ST-segment elevation MI. All patients received aspirin and were randomized to treatment with either unfractionated heparin or tirofiban, given as a loading dose of 0.6 µg/kg/min over 30 minutes followed by a maintenance infusion of 0.15 µg/kg/min for 48 hours (angiography/revascularization was discouraged during the infusion period). The primary composite end point (death, MI, refractory ischemia) at 48 hours was 5.6% in tirofiban-treated patients and 3.8% in placebo (aspirin/heparin)- treated patients (risk reduction 33%). Benefit was maintained but overall was less impressive at 7 and 30 days.

The PRISM in Patients Limited by Unstable Signs and Symptoms (PLUS) trial[13] included 1915 patients with unstable angina and non–ST-segment elevation MI who were treated with aspirin and heparin and randomized to either tirofiban (0.4 µg/kg/min x 30 min; then 0.1 µg/kg/min for a minimum of 48 hours and a maximum of 108 hours) or placebo (unfractionated heparin). Angiography and revascularization were performed at the discretion of the treating physician. Tirofiban-treated patients had a lower composite event rate of 7 days than the placebo group, 12.9% vs 17.9%, risk reduction 34%. The benefit was mainly due to a reduced incidence of MI (47% risk reduction) and refractory ischemia (30% risk reduction). The benefit was maintained at 30 days (22% risk reduction in composite event rate) and at 6 months (Table 8.2). The trial originally included a tirofiban alone arm (no heparin) that was dropped because of excess mortality at 7 days.

The importance of early intervention among patients with non–ST-segment elevation acute coronary syndromes was emphasized in the Treat Angina With Aggrastat and Determine Cost of Therapy With an Invasive or Conservative Strategy (TACTICS)–Thrombolysis in Myocardial Infarction (TIMI) 18 trial,[14] as was the benefit of aggressive pharmacologic therapy (GPIIb/IIIa receptor antagonists) in combination with PCI for patients at greatest risk for adverse ischemic outcomes (prior MI, ST-segment changes, elevated cardiac enzymes).

■ **Eptifibatide**

Eptifibatide (Integrilin) is a nonimmunogenic cyclic heptapeptide with an active pharmacophore that is derived from the structure of barbourin, a platelet GPIIb/IIIa inhibitor from the venom of the southeastern pigmy rattlesnake.[15]

TABLE 8.2 — CLINICAL TRIALS OF TIROFIBAN (AGGRASTAT): THE PRISM AND PRISM-PLUS STUDIES						
Events (%)	PRISM			PRISM-Plus		
	Tirofiban	Heparin	Risk Ratio	Tirofiban + Heparin	Heparin	Risk Ratio
48 Hours						
Composite	3.8	5.6	0.67*	7.8	5.7	0.71
Refractory ischemia	3.5	5.3	0.65*	4.8	5.9	0.78
MI or death	1.2	1.6	0.76	0.9	2.6	0.34*
MI	0.9	1.4	0.64	0.8	2.4	0.32*
Death	0.4	0.2	1.48	0.3	0.1	0.51
7 Days						
Composite	10.3	11.2	0.90	12.9	17.9	0.68*
Refractory ischemia	9.1	9.9	0.91	9.3	12.7	0.70*
MI or death	3.3	4.2	0.77	4.9	8.3	0.57*
MI	3.6	3.1	0.84	3.9	7.0	0.53*
Death	1.0	1.6	0.63	1.9	1.9	1.01
30 Days						
Composite	15.9	17.1	0.92	18.5	22.3	0.78*

Refractory ischemia	10.6	10.8	0.98	10.6	13.4	0.76
MI or death	5.8	7.1	0.80	8.7	11.9	0.70*
MI	4.1	4.3	0.95	6.6	9.2	0.70
Death	2.3	2.6	0.62*	3.6	4.5	0.79
6 Months						
Composite	—	—	—	27.7	32.1	0.81*
Refractory ischemia	—	—	—	10.6	13.4	0.76
MI or death	—	—	—	12.3	15.3	0.78
MI	—	—	—	8.3	10.5	0.76
Death	—	—	—	6.9	7.0	0.97
Readmission for unstable angina	—	—	—	10.9	10.7	1.00

Abbreviations: MI, myocardial infarction; PRISM, Platelet Receptor Inhibition in Ischemic Syndrome Management; PRISM-Plus, Platelet Receptor Inhibition in Ischemic Syndrome Management in Patients Limited by Unstable Signs and Symptoms.

* $P < 0.05$.

8

Pharmacokinetics

The plasma half-life of eptifibatide is 10 to 15 minutes and clearance is predominantly renal (75%) and to a lesser degree hepatic (25%). The antiplatelet effect has a rapid onset of action and is rapidly reversible.

Pharmacodynamics

In a pilot study of patients undergoing percutaneous coronary intervention (PCI), patients were randomized to one of four eptifibatide dosing schedules:

- 180 μg/kg bolus, 1 μg/kg/min infusion
- 135 μg/kg bolus, 0.5 μg/kg/min infusion
- 90 μg/kg bolus, 0.75 μg/kg/min infusion
- 135 μg/kg bolus, 0.75 μg/kg/min infusion.

All patients received aspirin and heparin and were continued on the study drug for 18 to 24 hours. The two highest bolus doses produced >80% inhibition of ADP-mediated platelet aggregation within 15 minutes of administration in a majority of patients (>75%). A constant infusion of 0.75 μg/kg/min maintained the antiplatelet effect, whereas an infusion of 0.50 μg/kg/min allowed gradual recovery of platelet function. In all dosing groups, platelet-function returned to >50% of baseline within 4 hours of terminating the infusion.[16]

Clinical Trials and Experience

The Integrilin to Minimize Platelet Aggregation and Coronary Thrombosis (IMPACT-II) trial[17] enrolled 4010 patients undergoing elective, urgent, or emergency coronary interventions. Patients were assigned to either placebo, a bolus of 135 μg/kg eptifibatide followed by an infusion of 0.5 μg/kg/min for 20 to 24 hours, or 135 μg/kg bolus with a 0.75 μg/kg/min infusion. By 30 days, the composite end point (death, MI, unplanned revascularization, stent placement for abrupt closure) occurred in 11.4%, 9.2%, and 9.9% of patients, respectively. Although the benefit of treatment was maintained at 6 months, the differences between groups were not statistically significant.

The IMPACT-After Myocardial Infarction (AMI) Study[18] was designed to determine the effect of eptifibatide on coronary arterial patency when used adjunctively with accelerated tissue plasminogen activator (tPA). A total of 132 patients with MI received tPA, heparin, and aspirin, and were randomized to receive a bolus and continuous infusion of one of six eptifibatide doses or placebo. The doses ranged from 36 to 180 µg/kg (bolus) to 0.2 to 0.75 µg/kg/min (infusion). Study drug was started within 30 minutes of tPA administration and continued for 24 hours. The highest dose eptifibatide groups had more complete reperfusion (TIMI Grade 3 flow) and shorter mean time to ST-segment recovery than placebo-treated patients. The composite clinical event rate (death, reinfarction, revascularization, heart failure, hypertension, stroke) was relatively high in all groups: 44.8% in eptifibatide-treated patients and 41.8% in placebo-treated patients.

The Platelet Glycoprotein IIb/IIIa in Unstable Angina Receptor Suppression Using Integrilin Therapy (PURSUIT) trial [19] included patients with unstable angina or non–ST-segment elevation MI with symptoms within 24 hours and electrocardiographic changes within 12 hours (of ischemia). A total of 10,948 patients were randomized to eptifibatide: 180 µg/kg bolus plus 1.3 µg/kg/min infusion, or 180 µg/kg bolus plus 2.0 µg/kg/min infusion or placebo for up to 3 days (in addition to heparin [in most patients] and aspirin). The 30-day event rate of death or nonfatal MI was 14.2% with eptifibatide and 15.7% with placebo (1.5% absolute reduction) (Figure 8.3). A reduction in MI or death (composite) with eptifibatide was observed at 96 hours, 7 days, and 30 days in medically or interventionally treated patients; however, the benefit was less impressive at later time points.

The Enhanced Suppression of the Platelet GPIIb/IIIa Receptor With Integrilin Trial (ESPRIT) was designed to test the hypothesis that a minimum threshold of 80% GPIIb/IIIa receptor blockade was required for benefit.[20] A total of 2064 patients received either eptifibatide (180 µg/kg boluses [x 2] 10 minutes apart, continuous infusion of 2.0 µg/kg/min for 18 to 24 hours) or placebo prior to PCI. The trial was terminated early for efficacy as patients receiving eptifibatide had a 4.0% absolute reduction in death, MI, urgent target vessel revascularization, or "bailout" GPIIb/IIIa antagonist use within 48 hours compared with placebo. Major events were significantly lower at 30 days as well.

8

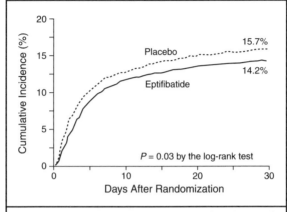

FIGURE 8.3 — INCIDENCE OF DEATH OR NONFATAL MYOCARDIAL INFARCTION ILLUSTRATED BY KAPLAN-MEIER CURVES

Kaplan-Meier curves showing the incidence of death or nonfatal myocardial infarction at 30 days. This analysis is based on end points as assessed by the central clinical events committee. The percentages shown are for the incidence at 30 days.

The PURSUIT Trial Investigators. *N Engl J Med.* 1998;339:436-443.

Similarities and Differences Between Intravenous GPIIb/IIIa Antagonists

Although considered collectively as GPIIb/IIIa receptor antagonists, abciximab, tirofiban, and eptifibatide differ at several levels, including their:

- Molecular size
- Binding characteristics
- Clearance
- Plasma
- Platelet-bound and biologic half-life
- Potential reversibility (Table 8.3).

The duration of platelet inhibition following drug discontinuation and the potential for reversing the pharmacologic effect are particularly important properties in cases of emergent surgery and major hemorrhagic complications. In general, a return of platelet function toward a physiologic state (≤50% inhibition) occurs within 4 hours following the cessation of tirofiban and eptifibatide. In contrast, 12 hours are required for abciximab (Figure 8.4). Some of the delayed return of physiologic platelet function following abciximab termination may be counterbalanced by its low free plasma concentration and drug-to-receptor ratio. These properties are responsible for the rapid return of hemostatic potential following platelet transfusions. In contrast, the high plasma concentrations observed with the small-molecule inhibitors limit the effectiveness of platelet transfusions. Fibrinogen supplementation (fresh frozen plasma, cryoprecipitate) is the more logical choice for restoration of hemostatic potential, given the competitive nature of binding and relative availability of platelet GPIIb/IIIa receptors[21] (Figure 8.5).

Major Clinical End Points

The intravenous GPIIb/IIIa receptor antagonists have been shown to reduce cardiac event rates in patients with acute coronary syndromes who are treated by pharmacologic means alone or undergo PCI. The available data suggest that the greatest overall benefit occurs in high-risk patients, many of whom require mechanical revascularization.

Methodologic differences between the major clinical trials make it difficult to compare the GPIIb/IIIa receptor antagonists; however, there is clear consistency among the agents with regard to efficacy and safety.[22] Meticulous attention to femoral arterial access, sheath care, and periprocedural heparin dosing has reduced vascular and major hemorrhagic complications substantially.

The Do Tirofiban And ReoPro Give Similar Efficacy Trial (TARGET) randomized 5308 patients to either tirofiban (RESTORE trial dosing strategy) or abciximab before PCI (with the intent to perform stenting). The primary end point, a composite of death, nonfatal MI, or urgent revascularization at 30 days, was reached in 7.6% and 6.0% of tirofiban-treated and abciximab-treated patients, respectively (hazard ratio 1.26).[23] There were no differences in the rates of major bleeding complications or transfusions,

TABLE 8.3 — INDIVIDUAL CHARACTERISTICS OF THE GPIIB/IIIA RECEPTOR ANTAGONISTS			
Characteristic	Abciximab	Eptifibatide	Tirofiban
Type	Antibody	Peptide	Nonpeptide
Molecular weight (daltons)	~50,000	~800	~500
Platelet-bound half-life	Long (h)	Short (s)	Short (s)
Plasma half-life	Short (min)	Extended (2 h)	Extended (2 h)
Drug-to-GPIIb/IIIa receptor ratio	1.5-2.0	250-2500	> 250
50% return of platelet function (without transfusion)	12 h	~ 4 h	~ 4 h
Abbreviation: GP, glycoprotein.			

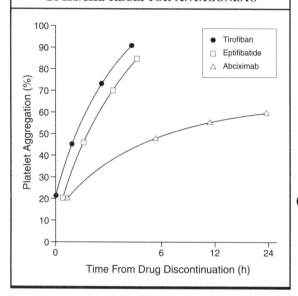

but tirofiban was associated with a lower rate of minor bleeding episodes and thrombocytopenia (Figure 8.6).

Thrombocytopenia

The administration of GPIIb/IIIa receptor antagonists is associated with thrombocytopenia (platelet count <100,000/mm^3) in approximately 2% to 3% of patients.[24] A more marked reduction (<50,000/mm^3) is seen in less than 1% of patients and may be influenced by:

- Concomitant procedures (coronary interventions)
- Medications (unfractionated heparin)
- Age (>65 years)
- Pretreatment platelet count
- Duration of treatment
- Repeat administration (even with a different agent than the first exposure).

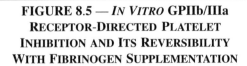

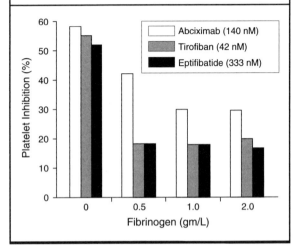

Acute, profound thrombocytopenia (<2000/mm³) has been reported within 4 hours of abciximab treatment.[25]

Oral GPIIb/IIIa Receptor Antagonists

The success enjoyed by intravenous GPIIb/IIIa receptor antagonists, coupled with the recognized risk for recurrent cardiac events incurred by patients with atherosclerotic coronary artery disease, stimulated interest in the development of oral agents that would provide continued, low-level GPIIb/IIIa receptor inhibition.

To date, over 30,000 patients have been enrolled in four large-scale, double-blind, placebo-controlled clinical trials. Individually, each trial failed to identify a reduction in ischemic outcomes. Collectively, a significant excess in mortality with three different oral GPIIb/IIIa antagonists was observed (Figure 8.7).[26]

FIGURE 8.6 — MAJOR CLINICAL OUTCOMES IN THE TARGET TRIAL

End Point	P	Hazard Ratio	Tirofiban (%)	Abciximab (%)
Composite	0.038		7.6	6.0
Death	0.66		0.5	0.4
Non-fatal MI	0.04		6.9	5.4
Death or non-fatal MI	0.04		7.2	5.7
Urgent target vessel revascularization	0.49		0.8	0.7

Hazard Ratio axis: 0.0 0.5 1.0 1.5 2.0 2.5 3.0 — Tirofiban Better / Abciximab Better

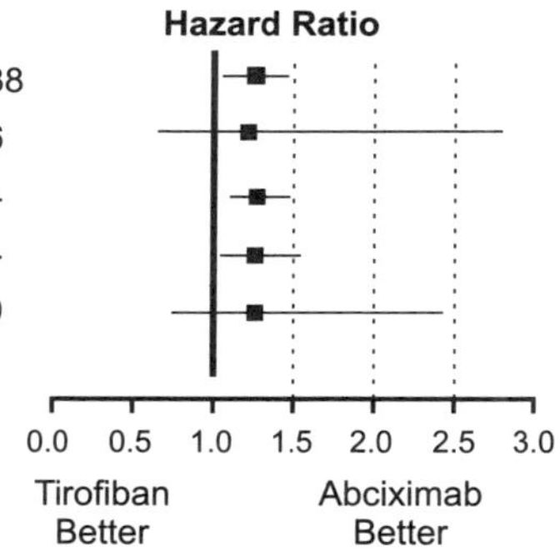

Abbreviation: MI, myocardial infarction.

Hazard ratios for the individual end points in Tirofiban and Give Similar Efficacy Outcomes Trial (TARGET).

Topol EJ, et al. N Engl J Med. 2001;34:1888-1894.

FIGURE 8.7 — MAJOR OUTCOMES IN TRIALS OF ORAL GPIIB/IIIA RECEPTOR ANTAGONISTS

Trial	No. in Study	Odds Ratio	Aspirin Alone (%)	GPIIb/IIIa Inhibitor (%)	P
EXCITE (xemilofiban)	7232	2.14	0.3	0.7	0.048
OPUS (orbofiban)	10288	1.40	1.4	2.0	0.049
SYMPHONY 1 (sibrafiban)	9169	1.14	1.8	2.0	0.420
SYMPHONY 2 (sibrafiban)	6637	1.55	1.3	2.1	0.038
Pooled	33,326	1.37	1.3	1.7	0.001

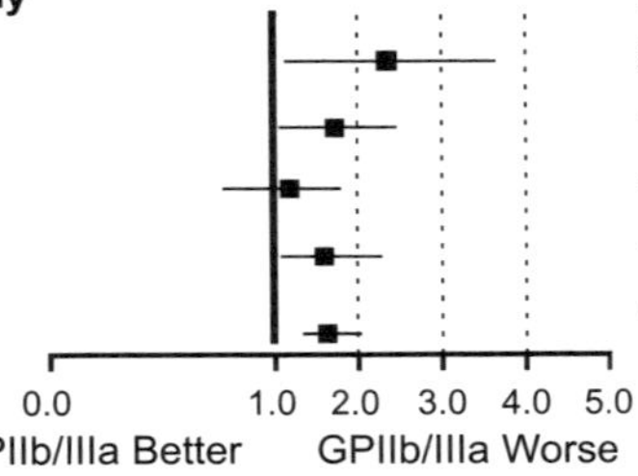

0.0   1.0 2.0 3.0 4.0 5.0

GPIIb/IIIa Better   GPIIb/IIIa Worse

Abbreviations: EXCITE, Evaluation of Oral Xemilofiban in Controlling Thrombotic Events, OPUS; Orbofiban in Patients With Unstable Coronary Syndromes; SYMPHONY, Sibrafiban vs Aspirin to Yield Maximum Protection From Ischemic Heart Events Post-acute Coronary Syndromes.

Odds ratio and 95% confidence intervals for death beyond 30 days in trials of oral GPIIb/IIIa receptor antgonists.

Chew DP, et al. *Circulation.* 2001;103:201-206.

Clinician's Approach to GPIIb/IIIa Antagonist Therapy

The wealth of available information allows several conclusions to be drawn regarding decision-making and patient care. First, the intravenous GPIIb/IIIa antagonists are an important component of medical and adjunctive therapy for acute coronary syndromes. Second, benefit is evident for both ST and non–ST elevation ischemic syndromes, particularly when combined with early PCI. Third, a threshold level of platelet inhibition must be achieved and maintained for maximum benefit. Fourth, combined pharmacotherapy with fibrinolytics requires further investigation to better define safe and effective dosing strategies, as will the role of facilitated PCI (Table 8.4). Fifth, the ideal comparative anticoagulant (low molecular weight heparin, very low molecular weight heparin, thrombin-directed antagonist, factor X inhibitor) and the potential non-platelet mediated beneficial effects, particularly as they relate to abciximab, must be determined through carefully designed trials. Last, future efforts in drug development must be mindful of pharmacokinetic and pharmacodynamic properties that may strongly influence dosing and overall clinical benefit.

8

Summary

The GPIIb/IIIa receptor represents a final common pathway for platelet aggregation. The development of GPIIb/IIIa receptor antagonists that can be administered intravenously represents a major step forward in the management of patients with acute coronary syndromes.

TABLE 8.4 — INTRAVENOUS GPIIB/IIIA RECEPTOR ANTAGONISTS: STRATEGIES FOR CLINICAL PRACTICE

Agent	Medical Treatment ACS	PCI	PCI STEMI	Fibrinolytic Combination STEMI	Facilitated PCI
Abciximab	++*	+++	+++	+	++
Eptifibatide	+++	+++	+	+	+
Tirofiban	+++	++	+	+	+

Key: +++, marked benefit; ++, moderate benefit; +, risk-benefit not fully defined.

Abbreviations: ACS, acute coronary syndrome; GP, glycoprotein; PCI, percutaneous coronary intervention; STEMI, ST elevation myocardial infartion.

* Refractory angina if PCI performed within 12 hours.

REFERENCES

1. Evaluation of Platelet IIb/IIIa Inhibition for Prevention of Ischemic Complications (EPIC) Investigators. Use of a monoclonal antibody directed against the platelet glycoprotein IIb/IIIa receptor in high-risk coronary angioplasty. *N Engl J Med*. 1994;330:956-961.

2. Topol EJ, Califf RM, Weisman HF, et al for the EPIC Investigators. Randomised trial of coronary intervention with antibody against platelet IIb/IIIa integrin for reduction of clinical restenosis: results at six months. *Lancet*. 1994;343:881-886.

3. Topol EJ, Ferguson JJ, Weisman HF, et al for the EPIC Investigator Group. Long-term protection from myocardial ischemic events in a randomized trial of brief integrin B_3 blockade with percutaneous coronary intervention. *JAMA*. 1997;278:479-484.

4. EPILOG Investigators. Platelet glycoprotein IIb/IIIa receptor blockade and low-dose heparin during percutaneous coronary revascularization. *N Engl J Med*. 1997;336:1689-1696.

5. CAPTURE Investigators. Randomized placebo-controlled trial of abciximab before and during coronary intervention in refractory unstable angina: the CAPTURE study. *Lancet*. 1997;349:1429-1435.

6. The GUSTO IV Investigators. Effect of glycoprotein IIb/IIIa receptor blocker abciximab on outcome in patients with acute coronary syndromes without early coronary revascularization: the GUSTO IV-ACS randomised trial. *Lancet*. 2001;357:1915-1924.

7. Montalescot G, Barragan P, Wittenberg O, et al, for the ADMIRAL Investigators. Platelet glycoprotein IIb/IIIa inhibition with coronary stenting for acute myocardial infarction. *N Engl J Med*. 2001;344: 1895-1903.

8. Gibson CM, de Lemos JA, Murphy SA, et al. Combination therapy with abciximab reduces angiographically evident thrombus in acute myocardial infarction: a TIMI 14 substudy. *Circulation*. 2001; 103:2550-2554.

9. Topol EJ, the GUSTO V Investigators. Reperfusion therapy for acute MI with fibrinolytic therapy or combination reduced fibrinolytic therapy and platelet glycoprotein IIb/IIIa inhibition: the GUSTO V randomised trial *Lancet*. 2001;357.1903-1914.

10. Kereiakes DJ, Kleiman NS, Ambrose J, et al. Randomized, double-blind, placebo-controlled dose-ranging study of tirofiban (MK-383) platelet IIb/IIIa blockade in high risk patients undergoing coronary angioplasty. *J Am Coll Cardiol*. 1996;27:536-542.

11. Randomized Efficacy Study of Tirofiban for Outcomes and Restenosis (RESTORE) Investigators. Effects of platelet glycoprotein IIb/IIIa blockade with tirofiban on adverse cardiac events in patients with unstable angina or acute myocardial infarction undergoing coronary angioplasty. *Circulation.* 1997;96:1445-1453.

12. Platelet Receptor Inhibition in Ischemic Syndrome Management (PRISM) Study Investigators. A comparison of aspirin plus tirofiban with aspirin plus heparin for unstable angina. *N Engl J Med.* 1998; 338:1498-1505.

13. Platelet Receptor Inhibition in Ischemic Syndrome Management in Patients Limited by Unstable Signs and Symptoms (PRISM PLUS) Study Investigators. Inhibition of the platelet glycoprotein IIb/IIIa receptor with tirofiban in unstable angina and non-Q wave myocardial infarction. *N Engl J Med.* 1998;338:1488-1497.

14. Cannon CP, Weintraub WS, Demopoulos LA, et al, for the TACTICS-TIMI 18 Investigators. Comparison of early invasive and conservative strategies for patients with unstable coronary syndromes treated with the glycoprotein IIb/IIIa inhibitor tirofiban. *N Engl J Med.* 2001;344:1879-1887.

15. Phillips DR, Scarborough RM. Clinical pharmacology of eptifibatide. *Am J Cardiol.* 1997;80:11B-20B.

16. Harrington RA, Kleiman NS, Kottke-Marchant K, et al. Immediate and reversible platelet inhibition after intravenous administration of a peptide glycoprotein IIb/IIIa inhibitor during percutaneous coronary intervention. *Am J Cardiol.* 1995;76:1222-1227.

17. Integrilin to Minimise Platelet Aggregation and Coronary Thrombosis (IMPACT)-II Investigators. Randomised placebo-controlled trial of effect of eptifibatide on complications of percutaneous coronary intervention: IMPACT-II. *Lancet.* 1997;349:1422-1428.

18. Ohman EM, Kleiman NS, Gacioch G, et al for the IMPACT-AMI Investigators. Combined accelerated tissue-plasminogen activator and platelet glycoprotein IIb/IIIa integrin receptor blockade with integrilin in acute myocardial infarction. Results of a randomized, placebo-controlled, dose-ranging trial. *Circulation.* 1997;95:846-854.

19. The Platelet Glycoprotein IIb/IIIa in Unstable Angina: Receptor Suppression Using Integrilin Therapy (PURSUIT) Trial Investigators. Inhibition of platelet glycoprotein IIb/IIIa with eptifibatide in patients with acute coronary syndromes. *N Engl J Med.* 1998;339:436-443.

20. The ESPRIT Investigators. Novel dosing regimen of eptifibatide in planned coronary stent implantation (ESPRIT): a randomised, placebo-controlled trial. *Lancet.* 2000;356:2037-2044.

21. Becker RC, Spencer FA, Liu T. Fibrinogen varying effects on GPIIb/IIIa receptor-directed platelet inhibition *in vitro. Am Heart J.* 2001;142:204-210.

22. Kong DF, Califf RM, Miller DP, et al. Clinical outcomes of therapeutic agents that block the platelet glycoprotein IIb/IIIa integrin in ischemic heart disease. *Circulation*. 1998;98:2829-2835.

23. Topol EJ, Moliterno DJ, Herrmann HC, et al, for the TARGET Investigators. Comparison of two platelet glycoprotein IIb/IIIa inhibitors, tirofiban and abciximab, for the prevention of ischemic events with percutaneous coronary revascularization. *N Engl J Med*. 2001; 344:1888-1894.

24. Giugliano RP. Drug-induced thrombocytopenia—is it a serious concern for glycoprotein IIb/IIIa receptor inhibitors? *J Thromb Thrombolysis*. 1998;5:191-202.

25. Berkowitz SD, Harrington RA, Rund MM, Tcheng JE. Acute profound thrombocytopenia after c7E3 Fab (abciximab) therapy. *Circulation*. 1997;95:809-813.

26. Chew DP, Bhatt DL, Sapp S, Topol EJ. Increased mortality with oral platelet glycoprotein IIb/IIIa antagonists. *Circulation*. 2001;103:201-206.

8

9   Monitoring of Anticoagulants

Introduction

Because of the narrow therapeutic index of warfarin and unfractionated heparin (UFH), monitoring of the anticoagulant effect of these drugs is required. On the other hand, low molecular weight heparin (LMWH) and fibrinolytic agents need to be monitored only under certain specific circumstances, to be described subsequently. Laboratory control of anticoagulants adds a level of complexity to treatment; variations in procedures and reagents can complicate management, especially if different laboratories are involved in the care of a single patient. Efforts to standardize testing must be an ongoing process as new methods and reagents are continually being introduced.

Warfarin

The prothrombin time is used to monitor warfarin treatment. This test is sensitive to the plasma concentrations of clotting factors II (prothrombin), V, VII, and X. Warfarin affects the vitamin K–dependent factors: II, VII, IX, and X, as well as proteins C, S, and Z. Thus the prothrombin time does not reflect the effect of warfarin on some factors (IX, proteins C, S, and Z) and is sensitive to others (factor V), which are not vitamin K–dependent. Therefore, the prothrombin time is not the ideal test of warfarin treatment, but its simplicity and widespread availability have enshrined it in clinical practice.

By convention, prothrombin times are now reported as international normalized ratio (INR). This is the ratio of the patient's prothrombin time to a control prothrombin time, raised to a power—the international sensitivity index (ISI). The latter reflects the calibration of the thromboplastin used for the prothrombin time testing to an internationally agreed upon standard. In many laboratories, the reagent currently used is a recombinant thromboplastin which has an ISI of

1, whereas in the past, the most commonly used reagents had ISIs of 2. In a laboratory with a control prothrombin time of 10 seconds, a prothrombin time of 15 seconds using a thromboplastin with ISI of 2 would have a calculated INR of 2.25 (15/10).[2] The same INR could be achieved with a recombinant thromboplastin (ISI of 1), but the prothrombin time would be 22.5 seconds (22.5/10).[1] Thus, the INR standardizes test values across laboratories using different reagents.

An INR in the range of 2 to 3 has been found to be optimal for patients with thrombotic disease; this was best exemplified in the Stroke Prevention in Atrial Fibrillation (SPAF) studies.[1,2] In these trials of oral anticoagulation in atrial fibrillation, INR values of less than 2 were most often associated with thrombotic events, while most hemorrhagic events occurred when the INR exceeded 3. Similar results have been obtained in patients with deep vein thrombosis and pulmonary embolism. INRs of 2 to 3 have also been recommended for the prevention of thromboembolism in patients undergoing high-risk surgery (joint replacement), and in those with valvular heart disease.[3] On the other hand, higher INRs have been suggested for patients with the lupus anticoagulant/antiphospholipid antibody (APA) syndrome and for those with prosthetic heart valves. With regard to the APA syndrome, retrospective studies indicated that INR values of 3 to 4 were more effective in thrombus prevention than lower ranges. However, prospective studies randomizing patients to INRs of 2 to 3 vs 3 to 4 are currently underway and should establish whether the higher range is necessary. Mechanical prosthetic heart values pose a high risk of thromboembolism. The recommendations of the Sixth American College of Chest Physicians (ACCP) Consensus Conference on Antithrombotic Therapy with regard to the various types of valves are summarized in Table 9.1.[4]

There are a few cautions in interpreting the results of prothrombin time tests.[5] Since the test is sensitive to the level of factor V in the plasma, improper sample storage or delayed testing may cause loss of factor V and give prothrombin time values outside the expected range. High concentrations of heparin may also prolong the prothrombin time; this usually occurs when the sample is obtained within

TABLE 9.1 — INTENSITY OF ORAL ANTICOAGULANT THERAPY IN PATIENTS WITH PROSTHETIC HEART VALVES (ACCP RECOMMENDATIONS)

Type of Valve	Location	Recommended INR
Mechanical		
Bileaflet	Aortic	2.0-3.0
Bileaflet with AF	Aortic	2.5-3.5 or 2.0-3.0 plus ASA 80-100 mg/day
Bileaflet	Mitral	2.5-3.5 or 2.0-3.0 plus ASA 80-100 mg/day
Tilting disk	Mitral	2.5-3.5 or 2.0-3.0 plus ASA 80-100 mg/day
Caged ball	Any	2.5-3.5 plus ASA 80-100/day
Bioprosthetic		
No AF	Aortic/mitral	2.0-3.0: first 3 mo postop
AF, atrial thrombus, prior thromboembolismm	Aortic/mitral	2.0-3.0: indefinitely

Abbreviations: ACCP, American College of Chest Physicians; AF, atrial fibrillation; ASA, aspirin; INR, international normalized ratio.

Proceedings of the ACCP 6th Consensus Conference on Antithrombotic Therapy. *Chest.* 2001;119(suppl):220S-227S.

9

a few minutes of administering a bolus dose of heparin. Neutralizing heparin prior to sample testing may allow one to overcome this problem. Direct thrombin inhibitors, such as hirudin and argatroban, may also prolong the prothrombin time to a modest degree. Some thromboplastins are sensitive to the lupus anticoagulant; the prolonged prothrombin times reported under these circumstances may deceive the clinician into thinking that the patient is adequately anticoagulated. In patients known to have a lupus anticoagulant, prothrombin times should be performed with thromboplastins that are insensitive to lupus anticoagulant, or other tests, such as factor X assay, should be obtained.

Heparin

Unfractionated heparin is monitored with the activated partial thromboplastin time (aPTT) test. In contrast to the prothrombin time, there is no generally agreed upon standardization for the aPTT. Different laboratories use reagents with varying sensitivities to the effects of UFH. Therapeutic anticoagulation requires heparin concentrations of 0.2 to 0.4 U/mL; in most laboratories this would correspond to aPTT values 1.5 to 2.5 times control values. However, each laboratory should calibrate its particular aPTT reagents against plasma containing a known amount of heparin, usually measured by the protamine titration method.[6]

Studies by Hull and colleagues demonstrated the importance of rapidly achieving a therapeutic aPTT.[7] Patients whose aPTT failed to reach therapeutic levels by 24 hours after the start of therapy were at increased risk of subsequent recurrent venous thrombosis. Several methods for rapidly achieving therapeutic aPTTs have been published; these are summarized in Table 9.2.[8-10] Hull and associates[9] make an adjustment for clinical history of increased bleeding risk, and the nomogram of Raschke and colleagues[10] is based on body weight. All of the methods were successful in having the aPTTs of the majority of patients exceed the lower limit of the therapeutic range at 24 hours. However, bleeding occurred more frequently in patients managed with the Hull nomogram than in those treated according to the Raschke method. At our institution, we prefer the weight-based nomogram because of its simplicity, safety, and effectiveness.

TABLE 9.2 — REGIMENS USING UNFRACTIONATED HEPARIN FOR THE TREATMENT OF VENOUS THROMBOEMBOLISM

Cruikshank 5000 U* (1280 U/h)		Hull 5000 U* (1680 U/h); High Risk† = 1240 U/h		Raschke 80 U/kg* (18 U/kg/h)	
aPTT (s)	Rate Change (U/h)	aPTT (s)	Rate Change (U/h)	aPTT (s)	Rate Change (U/kg/h)
<50	+120	<45	+240	<35	+4
50-59	+120	46-54	+120	35-45	+2
60-85	0	55-85	0	46-70	0
86-95	–80	86-110	–120	71-90	–2
95-120	–80	>110	–240	>90	–3
>120	–160	—	—	—	—

Abbreviation: aPTT, activated partial thromboplastin time.

* Bolus followed by continuous infusion.
† Patients having surgery within past 2 weeks, history of peptic ulcer, gastrointestinal or genitourinary tract bleeding, thrombotic stroke within past 2 weeks, platelet count <150,000/ mL, high risk of bleeding.

Cruikshank MK, et al. *Arch Intern Med.* 1991;151:333-337; Hull RD, et al. *Arch Intern Med.* 1992;152:1589-1595; Raschke RA, et al. *Ann Intern Med.* 1993;119:874-881.

Low molecular weight heparin does not require laboratory monitoring in clinically stable patients, whether given for prophylaxis or treatment.[11] Monitoring is recommended in the following situations:

- Pediatric patients and in those who weigh less than 50 kg
- Patients weighing more than 120 kg
- Pregnant patients, initially and during the third trimester
- Patients with renal failure (creatinine >2 mg/dL)
- Patients at high risk for bleeding.

The usual test selected for monitoring is the chromogenic anti–factor Xa (anti-Xa) assay, obtained 4 hours after the dose of LMWH. Levine and colleagues studied patients receiving LMWH prophylaxis for hip replacement.[12] Wound hematoma occurred in 5.3% when the anti-Xa level was ≤0.2 U/mL, but increased to 24.5% when levels exceeded 0.2. Conversely, thrombosis was 6.3% if minimum anti-Xa levels exceeded 0.1 U/mL but increased to 14.6% when ≤0.1 U/mL. These differences were all statistically significant. One should recognize, however, that LMWHs have a variety of effects on hemostasis that are not assessed by the anti-Xa test; this measurement provides only an approximation of the antithrombotic activity of these agents. The anti-Xa assay in patients receiving therapeutic, as opposed to prophylactic, doses of the drug are much less predictive of bleeding or thrombosis. Values in excess of 1 U/mL appear to be associated with an increased risk of bleeding.

Direct Thrombin Inhibitors

Monitoring is required when the currently available direct thrombin inhibitors (lepirudin, bivalirudin, and argatroban) are administered.[11] Table 9.3 shows the tests that are used, the therapeutic range needed, and the conditions requiring dose adjustments for each agent. When lepirudin is used for cardiopulmonary bypass, the ecarin clotting time, titrated to the lepirudin plasma level, appears to be the most reliable monitoring assay. Levels of 3.5 to 4.5 U/mL are optimal.[13]

TABLE 9.3 — MONITORING DIRECT THROMBIN INHIBITORS

Agent	Test	Therapeutic Range	Dose Adjustment
Lepirudin	aPTT at 2 h*	1.5-2.5 (not to exceed 70s)	Renal failure
Bivalirudin	ACT at 45 min	300-350s[†]	Renal failure
Argatroban	aPTT at 2 h	1.5-3.0 (not to exceed 100s)	Liver failure

Abbreviations: ACT, activated clotting time; aPTT, activated partial thromboplastin time.

* Ecarin clotting time at 15 minute intervals for cardiopulmonary bypass.
† During percutaneous coronary intervention.

9

137

Fibrinolytic Agents

Monitoring plays a limited role in the management of thrombolytic therapy. Prior to initiating fibrinolytics, a careful clinical assessment should be conducted to evaluate the potential for serious bleeding. Hemorrhagic stroke or ischemic stroke within the past year, intracranial neoplasm, aortic dissection, recent surgery or trauma (<2 to 4 weeks), pregnancy, and active peptic ulcer are some of the conditions which would preclude thrombolysis except under the most dire circumstances.[14] Obtaining baseline tests of hemostasis such as a platelet count, aPTT, prothrombin time, thrombin time, and fibrinogen level, will detect underlying hemostatic abnormalities.[15]

To assess the systemic effects of therapy, the reduction in fibrinogen, generation of fibrin degradation products, or depletion of plasminogen or α_2-antiplasmin may be examined.[16] If signs of excessive bleeding or oozing become apparent, measuring the fibrinogen level is helpful; values of less than 100 mg/dL may be associated with increased hemorrhagic risk.[17]

REFERENCES

1. Stroke Prevention in Atrial Fibrillation (SPAF) Investigators. Bleeding during antithrombotic therapy in patients with atrial fibrillation. *Arch Intern Med.* 1996;156:409-416.

2. Stroke Prevention in Atrial Fibrillation (SPAF) Investigators. Adjusted-dose warfarin versus low-intensity, fixed-dose warfarin plus aspirin for high-risk patients with atrial fibrillation: Stroke Prevention in Atrial Fibrillation III randomised clinical trial. *Lancet.* 1996;348:633-638.

3. Hirsh J, Dalen JE, Anderson DR, et al. Oral anticoagulants: mechanism of action, clinical effectiveness, and optimal therapeutic range. *Chest.* 1998;114(suppl):445S-469S.

4. Stein PD, Alpert JS, Dalen JE, Horstkotte D, Turpie AG. Antithrombotic therapy in patients with mechanical and biological prosthetic heart valves. *Chest.* 1998;114(suppl):602S-610S.

5. Fairweather RB, Ansell J, van den Besselaar MHP, et al. College of American Pathologists Conference XXXI on laboratory monitoring of oral anticoagulant therapy. *Arch Pathol Lab Med.* 1998;122:768-781.

6. Brill-Edwards P, Ginsberg JS, Johnston M, Hirsh J. Establishing a therapeutic range for heparin therapy. *Ann Intern Med.* 1993;119: 104-109.

7. Hull RD, Raskob GE, Brant RF, Pineo GF, Valentine KA. Relation between the time to achieve the lower limit of the aPTT therapeutic range and recurrent venous thromboembolism during heparin treatment for deep vein thrombosis. *Arch Intern Med.* 1997;157:2562-2568.

8. Cruikshank MK, Levine MN, Hirsh J, Roberts R, Siguenza M. A standard heparin nomogram for the management of heparin therapy. *Arch Intern Med.* 1991;151:333-337.

9. Hull RD, Raskob GE, Rosenbloom DR, et al. Optimal therapeutic level of heparin therapy in patients with venous thrombosis. *Arch Intern Med.* 1992;152:1589-1595.

10. Raschke RA, Reilly BM, Guidry JR, Fontana JR, Srinivas S. The weight-based heparin dosing nomogram compared with a "standard care" nomogram. *Ann Intern Med.* 1993;119:874-881.

11. Laposata M, Green D, Van Cott EM, Barrowcliffe TW, Goodnight SH, Sosolik RC. The clinical use and laboratory monitoring of low-molecular-weight heparin, danaparoid, hirudin and related compounds, and argatroban. *Arch Pathol Lab Med.* 1998;122:799-807.

12. Levine MN, Planes A, Hirsh J, Goodyear M, Vochelle N, Gent M. The relationship between anti-factor Xa level and clinical outcome in patients receiving enoxaparin low molecular weight heparin to prevent deep vein thrombosis after hip replacement. *Thromb Haemost.* 1989;62:940-944.

13. Poetzsch B, Madlener K. Management of cardiopulmonary bypass anticoagulation in patients with heparin-induced thrombocytopenia. in: Warkentin TE, Greinacher A, eds. *Heparin-Induced Thrombocytopenia.* New York: Marcel Dekker; 2000:355-369.

14. Leopold JA, Keaney JF Jr, Loscalzo J. Pharmacology of thrombolytic agents. In: Loscalzo J, Schafer AI, eds. *Thrombosis and Hemorrhage.* 2nd ed. Baltimore, Md: Williams & Wilkins; 1998:1236.

15. van Breda A, Katzen BT. Radiologic aspects of intra-arterial thrombolytic therapy. In: Comerota AJ, ed. *Thrombolytic Therapy.* Orlando, Fla: Grune & Stratton; 1988:113.

16. Nora RE, Bell WR. Practical aspects of thrombolytic therapy for deep vein thrombosis. In: Comerota AJ, ed. *Thrombolytic Therapy.* Orlando, Fla: Grune & Stratton; 1988:35-36.

17. Loscalzo J. Fibrinolytic therapy. In: Beutler E, Lichtmann MA, Coller BS, Kipps TJ, eds. *Williams Hematology.* 5th ed. New York, NY: McGraw-Hill, Inc; 1995:1389.

9

18. Comerota AJ. Complications of thrombolytic therapy. In: Comerota AJ, ed. *Thrombolytic Therapy*. Orlando, Fla: Grune & Stratton; 1988:266.

10   Monitoring of Platelet Activity

Despite the well-recognized benefits of platelet inhibition for the prevention and treatment of acute coronary syndromes, studies using traditional monitoring tools have not successfully achieved "proof of concept" in determining the degree of inhibition that is both safe and effective. In addition, measurements that are capable of assessing underlying atherosclerotic disease activity, prothrombotic potential, and response to treatment have not been developed for routine daily practice. The advent of near-patient assays and point-of-care technology may change management substantially, facilitating a more targeted and comprehensive approach.

Assessing Hemostatic Potential

Traditionally, platelet function studies have been employed in the evaluation of patients with unexplained bleeding where they have contributed greatly to the diagnosis and management of hereditary abnormalities such as von Willebrand disease, Glanzmann's thrombasthenia (platelet glycoprotein [GP] IIb/IIIa receptor deficiency) and Bernard-Soulier disease (platelet GPIb/IX receptor deficiency). Although conventional platelet function studies (turbidometric aggregometry) have technical limitations that preclude their routine use for gauging antithrombotic therapy, they may provide guidance when hemorrhagic complications arise and in determining pretreatment risk in individuals suspected of having an intrinsic platelet abnormality.

Bleeding Time

The bleeding time, considered an indicator of primary hemostasis (platelet plug formation), is defined as the time between making a small standardized skin incision and the precise moment when bleeding stops. The test is performed with a template, through which the medial surface of the forearm is incised under 40 mm Hg standard pressure. A normal bleeding time is between 6 and 10 minutes. Although considered a "standardized" test of platelet function, the bleeding time can be influenced by a variety of factors, including platelet count, qualitative abnormalities, and features intrinsic to the blood vessel wall.[1]

Platelet Adhesion Tests

Platelet adhesion is the initiating step in primary hemostasis. Although platelet binding is an important component of this process, there are many others, including blood flow rate, endothelial cell function, adhesive proteins, and the subendothelial matrix. The original platelet adhesion (or platelet retention) test was based on adherence to glass bead columns.

Platelet Aggregometry

The current laboratory evaluation of platelet function is based predominantly on *turbidometric platelet aggregometry* (also known as light transmission aggregometry). This test is performed by preparing platelet-rich plasma (with platelet-poor plasma as a control) and eliciting an aggregation response with adenosine diphosphate, epinephrine, collagen, arachidonic acid, and ristocetin.[2]

Impedance platelet aggregometry[3] has been introduced as an alternative to turbidometric methods, with the potential physiologic advantage of using whole blood samples. The reproducibility of platelet aggregometry is influenced by a variety of factors that include:

- Concentration of sodium citrate in the collecting tubes
- Adjustment of the platelet count
- Storage time
- Stirring rate
- Temperature
- pH of the blood sample.

Hereditary (Congenital) Abnormalities Affecting Platelet Function

Abnormal platelet function (qualitative defect) is capable of causing clinical hemorrhage that, at times, can be life-threatening. The common congenital thrombocytopathies for which *in vitro* testing may be diagnostic are summarized in Table 10.1.

Acquired Platelet Defects

Quantitative or, more commonly, qualitative platelet abnormalities are encountered frequently in clinical practice and in most cases represent a desired effect from drug therapy (Figure 10.1). A variety of systemic disorders can also influence platelet function (Table 10.2).

Flow Cytometry

Although not routinely available, flow cytometry offers a wide range of diagnostic capabilities for determining hemostatic potential, thrombotic potential, and response to platelet-inhibiting therapies. Whole blood samples are used and must be processed rapidly to maintain the "physiologic" environment.[4-6]

Bedside Assays and Instruments

Bedside assays, near-patient testing, and point-of-care monitoring instruments are attractive for several reasons. First, they provide a rapid, reliable, and reproducible means to assess hemostatic potential and treatment response. Second, the techniques involved require minimal training, reagent handling, calibration, and physical space. Third, emerging technology will offer a full complement of coagulation and platelet tests that can be used for management in the home, ambulatory clinic, emergency department, angioplasty suite, coronary care unit, and operating room.[7]

TABLE 10.1 — HEREDITARY PLATELET DISORDERS

Disease	Genetic Transmission	Specific Deficiency	Defect/Effect	Diagnosis
Glanzmann's thrombasthenia	Autosomal recessive	GP IIb/IIIa	Inability to bind fibrinogen and thus form platelet-to-platelet bridges	BT prolonged; abnormal aggregation response with all agonists; normal aggregation with ristocetin
Storage pool disease	Autosomal recessive and dominant	Storage and release of platelet granules	Important proteins for activation and aggregation inaccessible	Impaired aggregation response to various agonists
Bernard Soulier disease	Autosomal recessive	GP Ib/IX	Missing ligand for vWf leads to inability of platelets to bind to subendothelium	BT may exceed 20 min; thrombocytopenia; abnormal aggregation response with ristocetin
von Willebrand disease	—	—	—	Reduced vWf antigen
Type I	Autosomal dominant	vWf-factor VIII	Decreased adhesion	Decreased response to RIPA; decreased ristocetin cofactor activity

Type	Inheritance	Qualitative defect		
Type IIa	Autosomal dominant in vWf	Qualitative defect	Decreased adhesion	Reduced vWf; high molecular weight multimers
Type IIb	Autosomal dominant	Increased affinity of vWf for GPIb/IX receptor	Decreased adhesion	Reduced vWf; high molecular weight multimers; ↑ RIPA at low levels*
Type III	Autosomal dominant	Very low or absent vWf	Decreased adhesion	Similar to type I; severe bleeding common
Platelet type or pseudo vWd	Autosomal dominant	vWf receptor	Enhanced avidity for vWf leads to platelet consumption and low plasma vWf	RIPA with patient's platelets and normal plasma reproduce the defect; this differentiates from type IIb vWd

Abbreviations: BT, bleeding time; GP, glycoprotein; RIPA, ristocetin-induced platelet aggregation; vWf, von Willebrand disease; vWf, von Willebrand's factor.

* Aggregation in response to very low concentrations of ristocetin (<0.6 mg/mL).

10

145

FIGURE 10.1 — PHARMACOLOGIC CONTROL OF THROMBUS FORMATION

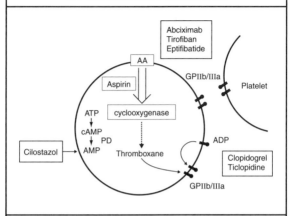

Abbreviations: AA, arachidonic acid; ADP, adenosine diphosphate; AMP, adenosine monophosphate; ATP, adenosine triphosphate; cAMP, cyclic adenosine monophosphate; GPIIb/IIIa, glycoprotein IIb/IIIa; PD, phosphodiesterase.

The available platelet antagonists "target" specific receptors and/or biologic events rendering the platelet "unfit" for participation in thrombus formation.

■ **Platelet Function Analyzer–100**

The platelet function analyzer (PFA)-100 simulates primary hemostasis under high shear stress conditions. Citrated whole blood is drawn by capillary action through a membrane coated with either collagen and epinephrine or collagen and adenosine diphosphate (ADP).[8] An aperature in the membrane occludes following platelet adhesion and aggregation and the test results are recorded as closure time.

The assay is most useful in detecting primary hemostasis abnormalities (primary platelet function disorders and von Willebrand disease) and determining response to replacement therapy.[9]

■ **Clot Retraction Assay**

The strength of clot retraction can serve as a measure of platelet function[10] and a hemostasis analyzer has been

TABLE 10.2 — ACQUIRED DEFECTS IN PLATELET FUNCTION

Drugs
- Aspirin
- Ticlopidine
- Clopidogrel
- Cilostazol
- Glyprotein (GP)IIb/IIIb antagonists (abciximab, tirofiban, eptifibatide)

Systemic Disorders and Disease States
- Chronic renal failure
- Myeloproliferative disorders
- Paraproteinemias
- Cardiopulmonary bypass
- Hemodialysis
- Disseminated intravascular coagulation

developed for this purpose. Citrated whole blood or platelet rich plasma is placed in a sample chamber where calcium and thrombin are added to stimulate clot formation. As platelets bind, undergo cellular contraction, and polymerize with fibrin strands, the force developed by the platelets is measured by a probe transducer that produces an electrical output (a voltage signal converted to force reported in dynes) proportional to the amount of force generated.

The clot retraction assay provides information on the functional contribution of platelets to clot formation, and can use whole blood or plasma obtained from standard citrated blood collection tubes. Potential uses include the evaluation of hemostatic defects in uremia and following bypass surgery.[11]

■ Rapid Platelet Function Assay

The Rapid Platelet Function Assay is a semi-automated turbidometric system that is based on the ability of activated platelets to interact with fibrinogen, yielding macroscopically visible agglutination.

Fibrinogen-coated polystyrene beads, buffers, and a modified thrombin receptor activating peptide (iso-TRAP) are incorporated into a disposable cartridge and exposed to samples of citrated whole blood. The instrument detects agglutination between the fibrinogen-coated beads and activated platelets, providing a quantitative digital display. Because agglutination is proportional to the proportion of unblocked GPIIb/IIIa receptors, this device is well suited for determining platelet inhibitory response to currently available GPIIb/IIIa receptor antagonists (Figure 10.2).[12] The time required to obtain results is 2 minutes.

The semi-automated system is easy to use and correlates closely with traditional measurements of platelet function, turbidometric platelet aggregation ($r^2 = 0.95$) and the percentage of free GPIIb/IIIa molecules ($r^2 = 0.96$).[13] The use of whole blood and duplicate analysis eliminates variables in sample preparation and minimizes random errors. Results can be reported as an absolute rate of aggregation or as a percentage of the baseline aggregation.

A rapid bedside assay that provides a reliable measurement of GPIIb/IIIa receptor blockade offers a broad range of medical, interventional, and surgical applications. Dose titration with intravenous agents could be performed, achieving a safe and effective degree of platelet inhibition.[14]

The intensity or level of platelet inhibition (achieved with GPIIb/IIIa antagonist therapy) required to prevent thrombotic complications following percutaneous coronary intervention (PCI) was determined in 485 patients participating in the GOLD study.[15] One quarter of all patients did not achieve $\geq 95\%$ inhibition (rapid platelet function assay) 10 minutes after the initiation of treatment and experienced a significantly higher incidence of death, myocardial infarction (MI), or urgent target vessel revascularization (14.4% versus 6.4%). Those with <70% inhibition at 8 hours were also at increased risk (25% versus 8.1%) (Figures 10.3 and 10.4).

A reliable and readily available means to assess inhibitory response to GPIIb/IIIa receptor antagonists may also provide guidance for dose titration in patients at risk for bleeding complications including those with thrombocytopenia, prior hemorrhagic events, and known coagulopathies (Table 10.3).[16]

FIGURE 10.2 — CORRELATION OF ABSOLUTE RATE OF PLATELET AGGREGATION WITH PERCENT AGGREGATION AT VARIOUS TIME POINTS FOLLOWING START OF ABCIXIMAB THERAPY

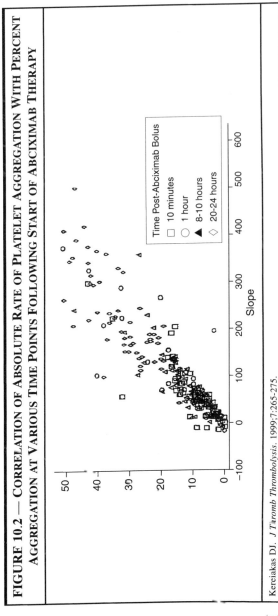

Kereiakas DJ. *J Thromb Thrombolysis.* 1999;7:265-275.

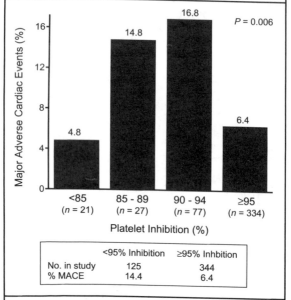

FIGURE 10.3 — ASSOCIATION BETWEEN EARLY GPIIB/IIIA ANTAGONIST-MEDIATED PLATELET INHIBITION AND CLINICAL EVENTS FOLLOWING PERCUTANEOUS CORONARY INTERVENTION

	<95% Inhibition	≥95% Inhbition
No. in study	125	344
% MACE	14.4	6.4

The occurrence of major adverse cardiac events (MACE), death, myocardial infarction, and urgent target vessel revascularization, correlated with the intensity of platelet inhibition 10 minutes after initiation of GPIIb/IIIa antagonist therapy.

Steinhubl SR, et al. *Circulation.* 2001;103:2572-2578.

Summary

The recognized role of platelets as the initiating step in arterial thrombosis provides a strong basis for their targeted inhibition in the primary and secondary prevention of cardiovascular events. Traditionally, the assessment of platelet activity has been viewed as a diagnostic tool for evaluating patients with hemorrhage. The development of

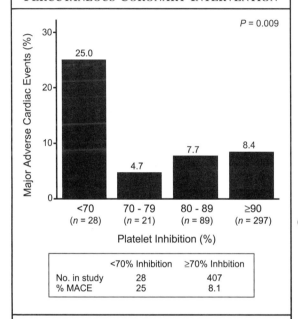

FIGURE 10.4 — THE THRESHOLD LEVEL OF PLATELET INHIBITION REQUIRED TO ACHIEVE OPTIMAL OUTCOME WITH GPIIb/IIIA RECEPTOR ANTAGONISTS IN PERCUTANEOUS CORONARY INTERVENTION

$P = 0.009$

	<70% Inhibition	≥70% Inhbition
No. in study	28	407
% MACE	25	8.1

In the GOLD study, major adverse cardiac events (MACE) correlated with the intensity of platelet inhibition 8 hours after initiation of treatment.

Steinhubl SR, et al. *Circulation*. 2001;103:2572-2578.

potent antagonists, coupled with a long-standing absence of information correlating treatment response, disease activity, and pharmacologic platelet inhibition, has fostered point-of-care technology that changes the focus of patient care from "one size fits all" to pathobiology-based, targeted antithrombotic intervention.

TABLE 10.3 — CLINICAL SETTINGS IN WHICH PLATELET MONITORING MIGHT BE USEFUL

Patient-Related (confirm target inhibition)
- Prior to percutaneous coronary intervention
- Patients with refractory ischemia or recurrent symptoms despite receiving glycoprotein (GP) IIb/IIIa receptor antagonist therapy
- Interruption of infusion
- Thrombocytopenia
- Qualitative platelet abnormality
- Renal insufficiency
- Low or high body weight

Clinically Related
- Bleeding:
  - Confirm intensity of inhibition
  - Confirm reversal of inhibition following replacement therapy
- Emergent surgery:
  - Guidance to reverse platelet inhibition (if clinically necessary)
- Transition from one GPIIb/IIIa receptor antagonist to another

REFERENCES

1. George JN, Shattil SJ. The clinical importance of acquired abnormalities of platelet function. *N Engl J Med.* 1991;324:27-39.

2. Born GVR. Qualitative investigations into the aggregation of blood platelets. *J Physiol* (London). 1962:67:162.

3. Cardinal DC, Flower RJ. The electronic aggregometer: a novel device for assessing platelet behavior in blood. *J Pharmacol Methods.* 1980;3:135-158.

4. Becker RC, Tracy RP, Bovill EG, Mann KG, Ault K for the TIMI-III Thrombosis and Anticoagulation Study Group. The clinical use of flow cytometry for assessing platelet activation in acute coronary syndromes. *Coronary Artery Dis.* 1994;5:339-345.

5. Becker RC, Bovill EG, Corrao JM, et al for the TIMI III Thrombo-sis and Coagulation Study Group. Platelet activation determined by flow cytometry persists despite antithrombotic therapy in patients with unstable angina and non-Q-wave myocardial infarction. *J Thromb Thrombolysis.* 1994;1:95-100.

6. Becker RC, Bovill EG, Corrao JM, et al. Dynamic nature of throm-bin generation, fibrin formation, and platelet activation in unstable angina and non-Q-wave myocardial infarction. *J Thromb Thromboly-sis.* 1995;2:57-64.

7. Becker RC. Exploring the medical need for alternate site testing. A clinician's perspective. *Arch Pathol Lab Med.* 1995;119:894-897.

8. Mammen EF, Comp PC, Gosselin R, et al. PFA-100 system: a new method for assessment of platelet dysfunction. *Semin Thromb Hemost.* 1998;24:195-202.

9. Jennings LK, White MM. Expression of ligand induced binding sites on glycoprotein IIb/IIIa complexes and the effect of various inhibi-tors. *Am Heart J.* 1998;135:S179-S183.

10. Greilich PE, Carr ME, Carr SL, Chang AS. Reductions in platelet force development by cardiopulmonary bypass are associated with hemorrhage. *Anesth Analg.* 1995;80:459-465.

11. Carr ME, Zekert SL, Hantgan RR, Braaten J. Glycoprotein IIb/IIIa blockade inhibits platelet-mediated force development and reduces gell elastic modulus. *Thromb Haemost.* 1995;73:499-505.

12. Coller BS, Scudder LE, Beer J, et al. Monoclonal antibodies to plate-let glycoprotein IIb/IIIa as antithrombotic agents. *Ann NY Acad Sci.* 1991;614:193-213.

13. Smith JW, Steinhubl SR, Lincoff AM, et al. Rapid platelet-function assay: an automated and quantitative cartridge-based method. *Cir-culation.* 1999;99:620-625.

14. Kereiakes DJ, Mueller M, Howard W, et al. Efficacy of abciximab induced platelet blockade using a rapid point of care assay. *J Thromb Thrombolysis.* 1999;7:265-276.

15. Steinhubl SR, Talley JD, Braden GA, et al. Point-of-care measured platelet inhibition correlates with a reduced risk of an adverse car-diac event after percutaneous coronary intervention: results of the GOLD (AU-Assessing Ultegra) multicenter study. *Circulation.* 2001;103:2572-2578.

16. Mukherjee D, Chew DP, Robbins M, et al. Clinical application of procedural platelet monitoring during percutaneous coronary inter-vention among patients at increased bleeding risk. *J Thromb Throm-bolysis.* 2001;11:151-154.

11 Inherited/Acquired Coagulation and Platelet Disorders (Thrombophilia)

Introduction

Thrombophilia is the term used to describe a tendency toward developing thrombosis. This tendency may be inherited, involving polymorphisms in gene coding for platelet or clotting factor proteins, or acquired due to alterations in the constituents of the blood or blood vessels. An example of a thrombophilic state that is both inherited and acquired is hyperhomocysteinemia; persons may have a genetic mutation leading to a modest defect in homocysteine metabolism, as well as a diet deficient in folate, with both contributing to an increase in plasma homocysteine and thrombosis.

When to Investigate for Thrombophilia

A complete history and physical examination are mandatory in patients presenting with either venous or arterial thrombosis. Inherited thrombophilia is likely if there is a history of repeated episodes of thrombosis or a family history of thromboembolism. One should also consider an inherited thrombophilia when there are no obvious predisposing factors for thrombosis or when clots occur in a patient under the age of 45. Repeated episodes of thromboembolism occurring in patients over the age of 45 raise suspicion of an occult malignancy. On the other hand, deep vein thrombosis (DVT) complicating joint replacement surgery occurs in persons without other risk factors, and a search for inherited thrombophilia usually is not warranted. Recurrence or extension of thrombus in a leg previously affected by DVT often indicates permanent damage to the involved venous structures and is a manifestation of the postphlebitic syndrome.

Inherited Thrombophilia

Some causes of inherited thrombophilia are shown in Table 11.1. This list is by no means complete, as new genetic polymorphisms are regularly being discovered and linked to a tendency to venous or arterial thrombosis.

Incidence

The prevalence of the more common thrombophilias is shown in Figure 11.1. Note that the factor V Leiden (FVL) mutation and hyperhomocysteinemia are present in nearly 5% of the general population and are often found in patients with venous thrombosis, while deficiencies of antithrombin (AT), protein C (PC), and protein S (PS) are relatively uncommon. Elevated levels of factor VIII (FVIII) are frequently noted in the general population and in patients with thrombosis. This is not surprising as FVIII is an acute-phase reactant that increases rapidly after surgery or trauma. However, prospective studies have shown that the increases in FVIII in some patients cannot be attributed to a stress reaction and probably indicate mutations in the genes controlling FVIII synthesis or release.[1]

The relative risks for thrombosis in patients with inherited thrombophilia have been examined. While AT mutations are the least common, they are associated with high frequencies of venous thrombosis (8%); similar risk is seen with PC and PS deficiency. In contrast, the lifetime risk of having a thromboembolic event in an individual heterozygous for FVL is only 2.2%.[2] Incidence rates markedly increase with age,[3] and are highest in those with AT deficiency, then PC and PS, and least with FVL.[4] FVL occurs with the highest frequency in persons of Northern European ancestry (3% to 8%), followed by Southern European (0.6% to 2.9%), and is rare in Asians and Africans. In the United States, the prevalence is 4% to 6%.[5]

Etiology

Mutations in the genes for either clotting factors or their inhibitors may increase the risk of thrombosis. A gene

TABLE 11.1 — CAUSES OF THROMBOPHILIA

Inherited
- Factor V Leiden mutation
- Prothrombin 20210A mutation
- MTHFR 677, CS mutations
- Mutations in protein C gene
- Mutations in protein S gene
- Mutations in antithrombin gene
- Mutations in TM and TFPI genes
- Increased FVIII, IX, X, ?vWF
- Mutations in fibrinogen genes
- Mutations in plasminogen gene
- Platelet GP1A mutation
- Increased PAI-1
- Mutant heparin cofactor II

Acquired
- Hyperhomocysteinemia
- Antiphospholipid antibody
- Pregnancy, estrogens, oral contraceptives
- Hyperlipidemias
- Nephrotic syndrome
- Malignancy
- Trauma
- Immobilization
- Myeloproliferative disorders
- Thrombotic microangiopathies
- Heparin-induced thrombocytopenia
- Endotoxemia

Abbreviations: GP, glycoprotein; PAI, plasminogen activator inhibitor; TFPI, tissue factor pathway inhibitor; TM, thrombomodulin; vWf, von Willebrand factor.

11

mutation may result In Increased production of a procoagulant protein, such as FVIII or prothrombin, or lead to a mutated factor that is resistant to inactivation by its natural inhibitor (factor V and activated protein C). An alteration in the amino acid sequence of antithrombin may prevent heparin from binding to and activating this anticoagulant. Mutant fibrinogens may be resistant to profibrinolytic

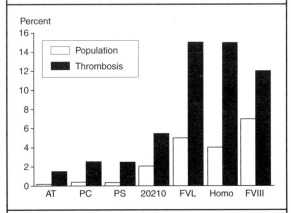

FIGURE 11.1 — PREVALENCE OF THROMBOPHILIA

Abbreviations: AT, antithrombin; FVIII, factor VIII; FVL, factor V Leiden; Homo, hyperhomocysteinemia; PC, protein C; PS, protein S; 20210, prothrombin 20210A.

Lensing AW et al. *Lancet.* 1999;353:479-485.

enzymes.[6] Lastly, patients may have more than one mutation, greatly increasing their risk of thrombosis.

Factor V Leiden is a mutant factor V that has an arginine to glutamic acid substitution at position 506, rendering the activated factor V partially resistant to inactivation by activated protein C (aPC).[7] The FVL also alters the ability of aPC to inactivate FVIII.[8] The impaired inactivation of activated factors V and VIII enhances blood coagulability. Persons may be either heterozygous or homozygous for the FVL mutation; thrombosis occurs much more frequently in those who are homozygous. In heterozygotes, the first episode of thrombosis usually occurs when there are superimposed risk factors such as surgery, trauma, immobilization, or exposure to oral contraceptives. The latter increases the risk of thrombosis more than fivefold.[9] Persistence of this trait in the population has been attributed to a decreased risk of intrapartum bleeding.[10] However, FVL is associated with recurrent fetal loss.[11,12] Other mutations in factor V may also contribute to the risk of thrombosis. For example, the

HR2 haplotype, a mutation predicting two amino acid changes is not in itself a risk factor for thrombosis. However, when coinherited with FVL, the risk of thrombosis is increased three- to fourfold.[13]

Prothrombin G20210A has a mutation in a regulatory sequence of the prothrombin gene leading to an increased synthesis of the prothrombin protein. Heterozygotes for the mutation have prothrombin concentrations that are increased about 1.3-fold,[14] and this is associated with an odds ratio of 2 to 3 for thrombosis.[15] An association of the prothrombin mutation with cerebral venous thrombosis has been reported.[16] As with FVL, there is also an increased frequency of thrombosis in women with this mutation who take oral contraceptives.[17]

Hyperhomocysteinemia may be congenital or acquired (Table 11.2).[18] In clinical practice, most patients with hyperhomocysteinemia are either homozygous for the C677T polymorphism of the MTHFP gene, and/or have nutritional folate deficiency. Thrombosis is associated with raised homocysteine levels but not the C677T mutation, and may occur in either the venous or arterial circulation. The usual manifestations are DVT, stroke, myocardial infarction (MI), and peripheral vascular disease. In one series, hyperhomocysteinemia was found in 13% of venous and 19% of arterial disease, and the risk for occlusive disease was increased 1.7 fold. Occlusive disease occurs at a younger age and there is a significantly higher recurrence rate.[19,20] Furthermore, the mortality associated with coronary heart disease is increased in proportion to the plasma homocysteine concentration.[21] The mechanism by which elevated levels of homocysteine promote thrombosis is unclear. There is experimental evidence of injury to the endothelium, decrease in nitric oxide (NO) production, induction of oxidation of low-density lipoprotein cholesterol, and increased affinity of lipoprotein (Lp) (a) for plasmin-modified fibrin surfaces, thereby inhibiting lysis of thrombi.[22-24] Plasma homocysteine concentrations decline when folate is taken, even in doses as low as 1 mg daily. In other patients, however, folate must be given along with vitamins B_6 and B_{12} in order to affect homocysteine levels. Clinical trials are in progress to determine whether a reduction in homocysteine levels actually alters thrombosis frequency.

TABLE 11.2 — CAUSES OF HYPERHOMOCYSTEINEMIA

- Genetic mutations:
  - Cystathione synthase
  - Methylenetetrahydrofolate reductase (MTHFR)
- Nutritional:
  - Deficiencies of folate, vitamin B_6, and vitamin B_{12}
- Diseases:
  - Kidney
  - Pernicious anemia
  - Hypothyroidism
  - Acute lymphocytic leukemia
  - Carcinoma of the breast, ovary, pancreas
  - Severe psoriasis
- Medications:
  - Folate antagonists
  - Oral contraceptives
  - Theophylline
- Miscellaneous:
  - Older age
  - Male sex
  - Menopause
  - Smoking

Adapted from Martinelli I, et al. *Arterioscler Thromb Vasc Biol.* 1999;19:700-703.

Proteins C, S, and AT are natural anticoagulant factors. Homozygosity for AT deficiency is lethal in utero, and for PC and PS, it leads to widespread thrombosis at birth (purpura fulminans) and death unless the protein is replaced by transfusion. Persons with one mutant gene (heterozygotes) develop thromboses in early adulthood, although some may not experience blood clots until later in life. Thrombi are usually venous in location and may affect mesenteric, cerebral, and other veins in addition to those in the legs and pelvis. In general, thrombosis occurs when there are risk factors in addition to the inherited mutations; these include surgery, cigarette smoking, pregnancy, and oral contraceptive use and any illness that results in bed rest, dehydration, and increases in stress-related proteins such as FVIII, fibrinogen, and plasminogen activator inhibitor-1.

Heparin cofactor II is a protease inhibitor like AT, but it is activated by dermatan sulfate rather than heparin. Thrombosis occurs only in persons with homozygous deficiency. Other causes of inherited thrombophilia include abnormalities in clot lysis. Cases have been reported where fibrin, the principal component of the blood clot, is altered so that it resists lysis, or there are mutations in the gene for plasminogen required for clot dissolution. Other components of the clotting pathway, such as thrombomodulin which is necessary for protein C activation, and tissue factor pathway inhibitor, an anticoagulant, may be abnormal and increase susceptibility to clotting.

Factor VIII has been found to be increased in one third of persons with thrombosis, as well as in their relatives, suggesting that mutations in the FVIII gene that give rise to increased FVIII activity will be important in thrombosis risk.[25] However, such mutations have not yet been discovered.[26] In addition, increased concentrations of fibrinogen and levels of factors IX and XI above the 90th percentile have been demonstrated to be risk factors for venous thrombosis.[27-29]

Location of Thrombi

In patients with inherited thrombophilia, thrombi are usually located in the venous circulation, with a few important exceptions. Patients with hyperhomocysteinemia may have early-onset arterial as well as venous thrombosis.[19] A study in Japan reported that the frequency of the MTHFR gene mutation (homozygous) was more than twice as high in stroke patients as in controls.[30] FVL and prothrombin 20210A are associated with a risk of MI in young women who smoke, and in male smokers, but not in nonsmokers.[31-33] The prothrombin mutation 20210A and FVL are both associated with an increased odds ratio for MI in male smokers, as well as in those with hypertension, hypercholesterolemia, and diabetes. The prothrombin mutation was also found to be overrepresented in persons who had a stroke prior to the age of 50.[34] As mentioned earlier, prothrombin 20210A is also associated with cerebral vein thrombosis. Inherited thrombophilia may lead to thrombosis of placental vessels. As previously noted, recurrent pregnancy losses occur in patients with FVL, and this is also the case for persons with the prothrombin mutation[35] and inherited deficiencies of AT, PC, and PS, and there is an eightfold risk of thrombosis in pregnancy.[36,37]

Platelet Abnormalities

A number of mutations in the genes controlling the formation of platelet proteins are being discovered; some of them may increase the tendency for thrombosis. For example, the platelet surface protein, glycoprotein (GP) Ia, mediates platelet binding to collagen, and GPIb mediates binding to von Willebrand's factor (vWf). Platelet GPIIb/IIIa is involved in the binding of fibrinogen. Mutations of these proteins (ie, GP1b and Pl^{A2}) have been implicated in increasing the risk for coronary heart disease and cerebral thrombosis.[38,39] A "sticky platelet" syndrome has also been described, associated with venous and arterial thrombosis.[40] There are likely many other platelet disorders predisposing to occlusive vascular disease.

Lastly, it should be emphasized that patients may have more than one risk factor; for example, heterozygosity for both FVL and prothrombin 20210A, or FVL and PS deficiency. Such combinations greatly increase the risk of thrombosis, as does homozygosity for FVL or the prothrombin mutation. In such cases, a history of thrombosis in family members is almost always obtained. Thrombosis risk is also greatly increased in the presence of other major risk factors such as cancer and diabetes. In these latter situations, thrombotic occlusion of coronary and cerebral arteries may occur in addition to venous thrombosis.

Acquired Thrombophilia

- **Acquired Deficiencies in Antithrombin, Protein C, and Protein S**
  Deficiencies of AT, PC, and PS may be acquired in the setting of a variety of disorders shown in Table 11.3. These three anticoagulant proteins are synthesized by the liver, and therefore levels are decreased when there is im-

162

TABLE 11.3 — ACQUIRED CAUSES OF ANTITHROMBIN, PROTEIN C, AND PROTEIN S DEFICIENCY		
Acquired Cause	Antithrombin	Protein C and Protein S
Synthesis	Prematurity, liver disease	Prematurity, liver disease, vitamin K deficiency
Excretion	Nephrotic syndrome, IBD	Nephrotic syndrome, IBD
Consumption	Disseminated intravascular coagulation, post-surgical, posttrauma	Disseminated intravascular coagulation
Medications	Heparin, estrogens, oral contraceptives, L-asparaginase	Warfarin, estrogens, oral contraceptives
Miscellaneous	Pregnancy	Pregnancy,* sickle cell disease,* antiphospholipid antibody syndrome, endotoxemia,* HIV infection*
Abbreviations: HIV, hur an immunodeficiency virus; IBD, inflammatory bowel disease.		
* Protein S deficiency.		

11

163

maturity or disease of the liver. In addition, PC and PS require vitamin K for completion of their synthesis; concentrations are reduced when there is vitamin K deficiency or when warfarin is administered. The three anticoagulants are lost in the urine in patients with nephrotic syndrome and in the stool of persons with protein-losing enteropathies. They are consumed when there is disseminated intravascular coagulation or extensive thrombosis. The metabolism of AT is similar to that of albumin; conditions resulting in decreases in albumin, such as major surgery or trauma, also lower AT concentrations, which may be a factor in the pathogenesis of postsurgical thrombosis. Heparin treatment results in a slight decrease in AT levels, while warfarin may cause significant declines in the concentrations of PC and PS, leading, in extreme cases, to thrombosis of cutaneous vessels and skin necrosis. Estrogens, oral contraceptives, and pregnancy are associated with lowering of AT and PS levels. A decrease in PS is a consistent finding in patients with sickle cell disease. Last, about two thirds of PS circulates bound to the C4b-binding protein; increases in this protein occur in endotoxemia and certain other infections, decreasing the availability of free PS. PC is decreased in patients undergoing marrow transplants who develop venoocclusive disease, and it is also reduced in those with the antiphospholipid antibody syndrome.

In addition, there are important acquired causes of resistance to activated protein C. These include pregnancy, oral contraceptives, oral anticoagulants, stroke, increased factor VIII levels, antiphospholipid antibody syndrome, and autoantibodies directed against activated protein C.[41] Patients with acquired protein C resistance are also susceptible to venous thrombosis; the greater the resistance, the higher the risk.[42]

■ Antiphospholipid Antibody Syndrome

Patients with this syndrome have a positive test for antibodies to phospholipid-protein complexes plus one of the following: venous or arterial thrombosis, livedo reticularis, neuropsychiatric disorder, valvular heart disease, thrombocytopenia, and/or recurrent fetal wastage.[43] The syndrome may be primary, meaning no associated disorders are present, or secondary to systemic lupus erythematosus, other autoimmune disorders, infections, malignancy, or exposure to certain drugs such as chlorpromazine, procainamide, or hydralazine. The diagnosis is based on the clinical findings of thrombosis, either arterial or venous, and a positive test for either anticardiolipin antibodies (ACA) (titer >40 GPL [IgG Phospholipid units]) or lupus anticoagulant. Antiphospholipid antibodies occur in about a third of patients with systemic lupus erythematosus but are also found in patients with rheumatoid arthritis, sickle cell disease, and in 10% to 15% of apparently healthy elderly individuals.[44]

Antiphospholipid-protein antibodies are a heterogeneous group of antibodies that recognize a variety of phospholipid-binding proteins; these include:

- $\beta_2$glycoprotein-1
- Prothrombin
- Clotting factors X and XI
- Proteins C and S
- Thrombomodulin
- Annexin V.

These antibodies are detected by ELISA assays that usually include anionic phospholipids such as cardiolipin (ACA) or coagulant phospholipids (LA). Goodnight[45] points out that the high titer (>40 GPL units) are more predictive of disease than low titer antibodies; antibodies directed against $\beta_2$glycoprotein-1 are more specific than IgM antibodies which may be markers for infection rather than thrombosis; LA are more associated with thrombosis than are ACA; and lastly, that multiple assays must be performed to assess patient risk for vascular disease.

The term "lupus anticoagulant" arose because the clotting times of phospholipid-based coagulation assays were prolonged by plasma from patients with lupus. This is because the antiphospholipid antibodies in the plasma of these patients interfere with the binding of clotting factors to procoagulant phospholipids. *In vivo*, however, these antibodies interfere with the binding of annexin V and $\beta_2$glycoprotein-1 to procoagulant phospholipids on cell membranes; this enhances the procoagulant activity of these membranes and is responsible for the thrombophilia.[46,47] In addition, antiphospholipid antibodies indirectly enhance the

165

binding of PS to its plasma inhibitor, the C4b-binding protein, by interfering with the protective effect of $\beta_2$glycoprotein-1 in maintaining free protein S.[48] Antibodies directed against activated protein C have also been associated with extensive arterial and venous thrombosis.[49]

Patients have either arterial disease (stroke, digital ischemia, retinal artery occlusion) or recurrent venous thrombosis. The LA is the strongest risk factor for both arterial and venous thrombosis, but ACA greater than 20 units is also an important risk factor for venous thrombosis.[50,51]

■ **Diagnosis**

An inherited thrombophilia is suspected in persons with thrombosis unexplained by obvious risk factors such as recent orthopedic, neurological, or other surgery or trauma. The diagnostic approach is shown in Table 11.4. A useful algorithm for deciding whether to perform extensive diagnostic studies for inherited thrombophilia is FURY: F refers to a positive family history, U to clotting at unusual sites, R to recurrent episodes of thrombosis, and Y to age under 45 (young). With regard to laboratory investigations, Seligsohn and Lubetsky recommend that a test for resistance to activated protein C be performed and, if positive,

---

TABLE 11.4 — DIAGNOSTIC APPROACH TO THROMBOPHILIA

- History: FURY
  - **F** = positive family history
  - **U** = clotting at unusual sites
  - **R** = recurrent episodes of thrombosis
  - **Y** = age under 45 (young)
- Laboratory studies:
  - aPC by clotting test: if positive, genetic analysis for factor V Leiden and factor V HR_2 mutation
  - Genetic analysis for prothrombin 20210 mutation
  - Lupus anticoagulant; anticardiolipin assay by enzyme-linked immunosorbent assay
  - Homocysteine
  - Antithrombin, proteins C and S (free and total)

Abbreviation: aPC, activated protein C.

---

followed by a genetic analysis for factor V Leiden and the HR$_2$ variant.[41] Other causes of activated protein C resistance include defects in proteins C or S, elevated levels of factor VIII, the use of oral contraceptives, and pregnancy. Further evaluation would include a test for the prothrombin G20210A mutation, screening for the lupus anticoagulant and anticardiolipin antibodies, and measurement of homocysteine concentration. The second tier of testing includes analysis of protein C, protein S, and antithrombin. Deficiencies or defects in these analytes are much less common and may be acutely affected by the thrombosis itself. Ordinarily, they should be measured at least 2 weeks after oral anticoagulant therapy has been completed when the effects of treatment and the acute phase of the illness have subsided. Should all of the above tests be unrevealing, further evaluation could include fibrinogen antigen and activity, measures of factors IX, XI, and polymorphisms of plasminogen and factor XIII.

■ Management

Thrombosis usually occurs in patients with more than one risk factor; if an inherited or acquired thrombophilia is present, oral contraceptives should be avoided, and prophylaxis against thrombosis should be given after surgery or trauma. The use of antithrombotic drugs is discussed in Chapter 3, *Heparin, Low Molecular Weight Heparin, Hirudin, and Warfarin*, but what is unique to the thrombophilic disorders is the duration and intensity of anticoagulant therapy. Venous thrombosis is usually treated with heparin or low molecular weight heparin (LMWH) and warfarin. When the international normalized ratio (INR) obtained by the prothrombin time test is in the range of 2 to 3 for at least 48 hours, the heparins are discontinued. Warfarin is then continued for varying time periods, depending on the perceived risk of recurrence of thrombosis. In patients with inherited thrombophilia, such as that caused by FVL, discontinuing treatment after 3 to 6 months is associated with a recurrence rate of almost 40% after 8 years, as compared with 18% in persons without this mutation.[52] Therefore, continuation of warfarin treatment for longer than 6 months may be considered but must be weighed against the risk of bleeding, which increases with each year of warfarin therapy.[53] In patients with the antiphospholipid antibody syndrome, elevated titers of ACA present 6 months after an episode of venous thromboembolism are predictive of an increased risk of recurrence, and therefore anticoagulants are usually continued indefinitely in such patients.[54]

A problem in the use of warfarin for management of patients with lupus anticoagulant (LA) is the confounding effect of this pathologic anticoagulant on the INR. Prolongation of the prothrombin time by the LA may be erroneously attributed to the warfarin, and result in inadequate dosing of the drug. This may be the reason why some retrospective studies suggested that increasing the intensity of warfarin treatment from an INR of 2 to 3 to an INR of 3 to 4 would be more effective in preventing recurrent episodes of thrombosis.[55,56] It might also be possible to monitor warfarin with a thromboplastin reagent that is insensitive to the LA or use a different assay method, but whether this strategy decreases thrombosis recurrence is still unclear. Because it is difficult to maintain the higher INR range and avoid bleeding, an alternative is to use the less intense 2-to-3 INR range, but supplement warfarin with small doses of aspirin, 81 mg daily. While there are theoretical advantages to this regimen, it has not been tested in formal clinical trials. In pregnant women with antiphospholipid antibody syndrome and a history of thrombosis, low-dose aspirin and heparin or LMWH must be given throughout pregnancy to prevent fetal loss as well as maternal thromboembolism.[57]

REFERENCES

1. Kamphuisen PW, Eikenboom JC, Vas HL, et al. Increased levels of factor VIII and fibrinogen in patients with venous thrombosis are not caused by acute phase reactions. *Thromb Haemost*. 1999;81:680-683.

2. Martinelli I, Mannucci PM, De Stefano V, et al. Different risks of thrombosis in four coagulation defects associated with inherited thrombophilia: a study of 150 families. *Blood*. 1998;92:2353-2358.

3. Ridker PM, Glynn RJ, Miletich JP, Goldhaber SZ, Stampfer MJ, Hennekens CH. Age-specific incidence rates of venous thromboembolism among heterozygous carriers of factor V Leiden mutation. *Ann Intern Med*. 1997:126:528-531.

4. Bucciarelli P, Rosendaal FR, Tripodi A, et al. Risk of venous thromboembolism and clinical manifestations in carriers of antithrombin, protein C, protein S deficiency, or activated protein C resistance. a multicenter collaborative family study. *Arterioscler Thromb Vasc Biol.* 1999;19:1026-1033.

5. Price DT, Ridker PM. Factor V Leiden mutation and the risks for thromboembolic disease: a clinical perspective. *Ann Intern Med.* 1997; 127:895-903.

6. Dang et al. Dysfibrinogenemias show decreased thrombin binding, absent plasmin degradation, decreased t-PA binding. *Am J Med.* 1989;87:567.

7. Dahlback B. Procoagulant and anticoagulant properties of coagulation factor V: factor V Leiden (APC resistance) causes hypercoagulability by dual mechanisms. *J Lab Clin Med.* 1999;133:415-422.

8. Tans G, Nicolaes GA, Rosing J. Regulation of thrombin formation by activated protein C: effect of the factor V Leiden mutation. *Semin Hematol.* 1997;34:244-255.

9. Vandenbroucke JP, Koster T, Briet E, Reitsma PH, Bertina RM, Rosendaal FR. Increased risk of venous thrombosis in oral-contraceptive users who are carriers of factor V Leiden mutation. *Lancet.* 1994;344:1453-1457.

10. Lindqvist PG, Svensson PJ, Dahlback B, Marsal K. Factor V Q^{506} mutation (activated protein C resistance) associated with reduced intrapartum blood loss—a possible evolutionary selection mechanism. *Thromb Haemost.* 1998;79:69-73.

11. Grandone E, Margaglione M, Colaizzo D, et al. Factor V Leiden is associated with repeated and recurrent unexplained fetal losses. *Thromb Haemost.* 1997;77:822-824.

12. Ridker PM, Miletich JP, Buring JE, et al. Factor V Leiden mutation as a risk factor for recurrent pregnancy loss. *Ann Intern Med.* 1998; 128:1000-1003.

13. Faioni EM, Franchi F, Bucciarelli P, et al. Coinheritance of the HR2 haplotype in the factor V gene confers an increased risk of venous thromboembolism to carriers of factor V R506Q (factor V Leiden). *Blood.* 1999;94:3062-3066.

14. Makris M, Preston FE, Beauchamp NJ, et al. Co-inheritance of the 20210A allele of the prothrombin gene increases the risk of thrombosis in subjects with familial thrombophilia. *Thromb Haemost.* 1997; 78:1426-1429.

15. van der Meer FJ, Koster T, Vandenbroucke JP, Briet E, Rosendaal FR. The Leiden Thrombophilia Study (LETS). *Thromb Haemost.* 1997;78:631-635.

169

16. Martinelli I, Sacchi E, Landi G, Taioli E, Duca F, Mannucci PM. High risk of cerebral-vein thrombosis in carriers of a prothrombin gene mutation and in users of oral contraceptives. *N Engl J Med.* 1998;338:1793-1797.

17. Martinelli I, Taioli E, Bucciarelli P, Akhavan S, Mannucci PM. Interaction between the G20210A mutation of the prothrombin gene and oral contraceptive use in deep vein thrombosis. *Arterioscler Thromb Vasc Biol.* 1999;19:700-703.

18. Hankey GJ, Eikelboom JW. Homocysteine and vascular disease. *Lancet.* 1999;354:407-413.

19. Fermo I, D'Angelo SV, Paroni R, Mazzola G, Calori G, D'Angelo A. Prevalence of moderate hyperhomocysteinemia in patients with early-onset venous and arterial occlusive disease. *Ann Intern Med.* 1995;123:747-753.

20. Eichinger S, Stumpflen A, Hirschl M, et al. Hyperhomocysteinemia is a risk factor of recurrent venous thromboembolism. *Thromb Haemost.* 1998;80:566-569.

21. Nygard O, Nordrehaug JE, Refsum H, Ueland PM, Farstad M, Vollset SE. Plasma homocysteine levels and mortality in patients with coronary artery disease. *N Engl J Med.* 1997;337:230-236.

22. Harpel PC, Chang VT, Borth W. Homocysteine and other sulfhydryl compounds enhance the binding of lipoprotein (a) to fibrin: a potential biochemical link between thrombosis, atherogenesis, and sulfhydryl compound metabolism. *Proc Natl Acad Sci USA.* 1992; 89:10193-10197.

23. D'Angelo A, Selhub J. Homocysteine and thrombotic disease. *Blood.* 1997;90:1-11.

24. Hajjar KA, Jacovina AT. Modulation of annexin II by homocysteine: implications for atherothrombosis. *J Investig Med.* 1998;46:364-369.

25. Schambeck CM, Hinney K, Haubitz I, Mansouri TB, Wahler D, Keller F. Familial clustering of high factor VIII levels in patients with venous thromboembolism. *Arterioscler Thromb Vasc Biol.* 2001;21:289-292.

26. Mansvelt EP, Laffan M, McVey JH, Tuddenham EG. Analysis of the F8 gene in individuals with high plasma factor VII:C levels and associated venous thrombosis. *Thromb Haemost.* 1998;80:561-565.

27. Koster T, Rosendaal FR, Reitsma PH, van der Velden PA, Briet E, Vandenbroucke JP. Factor VII and fibrinogen levels as risk factors for venous thrombosis: a case-control study of plasma levels and DNA polymorphisms—the Leiden Thrombophilia Study (LETS). *Thromb Haemost.* 1994;71:719-722.

28. van Hylckama Vlieg A, van der Linden IK, Vertina RM, Rosendaal FR. High levels of factor IX increase the risk of venous thrombosis. *Blood.* 2000;95:3678-3682.

29. Meijers JC, Tekelenburg WL, Bouma BN, Bertina RM, Rosendaal FR. High levels of coagulation fator XI as a risk factor for venous thrombosis. *N Engl J Med.* 2000;342:696-701.

30. Morita H, Kurihara H, Tsubaki S, et al. Methylenetetrahydrofolate reductase gene polymorphism and ischemic stroke in Japanese. *Arterioscler Thromb Vasc Biol.* 1998;18:1465-1469.

31. Rosendaal F, Siscovick DS, Schwartz SM, et al. Factor V Leiden (resistance to activated protein C) increases the risk of myocardial infarction in young women. *Blood.* 1997;89:2817-2821.

32. Rosendaal F, Siscovick DS, Schwartz SM, Psaty BM, Raghunathan TE, Vos HL. A common prothrombin variant (20210 G to A) increases the risk of myocardial infarction in young women. *Blood.* 1997;90:1747-1750.

33. Inbal A, Freimark D, Modan B, et al. Synergistic effects of prothrombotic polymorphisms and atherogenic factors on the risk of myocardial infarction in young males. *Blood.* 1999;93:2186-2190.

34. DeStefano V, Chiusolo P, Paciaroni K, et al. Prothrombin G20210A mutant genotype is a risk factor for cerebrovascular ischemic disease in young patients. *Blood.* 1998;91:3562-3565.

35. Martinelli I, Taioli E, Cetin I, et al. Mutations in coagulation factors in women with unexplained late fetal loss. *N Engl J Med.* 2000;343: 1015-1018.

36. Preston FE, Rosendaal FR, Walker ID, et al. Increased fetal loss in women with heritable thrombophilia. *Lancet.* 1996;348:913-916.

37. Friederich PW, Sanson BJ, Simioni P, et al. Frequency of pregnancy-related venous thromboembolism in anticoagulant factor-deficient women: implications for prophylaxis [published correction appears in *Ann Intern Med.* 1997;126:835 and 1997;127:1138]. *Ann Intern Med.* 1996;125:955-960.

38. Gonzalez-Conejero R, Lozano ML, Rivera J, et al. Polymorphisms of platelet membrane glycoprotein Ib associated with arterial thrombotic disease. *Blood.* 1998;92:2771-2776.

39. Weiss EJ, Bray PF, Tayback M, et al. A polymorphism of a platelet glycoprotein receptor as an inherited risk factor for coronary thrombosis. *N Engl J Med.* 1996;334:1090-1094.

40. Bick RL, Kaplan H. Syndromes of thrombosis and hypercoagulability. Congenital and acquired causes of thrombosis. *Med Clin North Am.* 1998;82:409-458.

41. Seligsohn U, Lubetsky A. Genetic susceptibility to venous thrombosis. *N Engl J Med*. 2001;344:1222-1231.

42. de Visser MC, Rosendaal FR, Bertina RM. A reduced sensitivity for activated protein C in the absence of factor V Leiden increases the risk of venous thrombosis. *Blood*. 1999;93:1271-1276.

43. Love PE, Santoro SA. Antiphospholipid antibodies: anticardiolipin and the lupus anticoagulant in systemic lupus erythematosus and in non-systemic lupus erythematosus disorders. Prevalence and clinical significance. *Ann Intern Med*. 1990;112:682-698.

44. Greaves M. Antiphospholipid antibodies and thrombosis. *Lancet*. 1999;353:1348-1353.

45. Goodnight SH. Antiphospholipid antibodies and thrombosis. In: McArthur JR, Schecter GP, eds. *Hematology 1998*. Washington, DC: American Society of Hematology; 1998:261-265.

46. Rand JH, Wu XX, Andree HA, et al. Antiphospholipid antibodies accelerate plasma coagulation by inhibiting annexin-V binding to phospholipids: a "lupus procoagulant" phenomenon. *Blood*. 1998;92:1652-1660.

47. Rand JH. "Annexinopathies"—a new class of diseases. *N Engl J Med*. 1999;340:1035-1036. Editorial.

48. Merrill JT, Zhang HW, Shen C, et al. Enhancement of protein S anticoagulant function by β_2-glycoprotein-1, a major target antigen of antiphospholipid antibodies. *Thromb Haemost*. 1999;81:748-757.

49. Zivelin A, Gitel S, Griffin JH, et al. Extensive venous and arterial thrombosis associated with an inhibitor to activated protein C. *Blood*. 1999;94:895-901.

50. Horbach DA, van Oort E, Donders RC, Derksen RH, de Groot PG. Lupus anticoagulant is the strongest risk factor for both venous and arterial thrombosis in patients with systemic lupus erythematosus. *Thromb Haemost*. 1996;76:916-924.

51. Ginsburg KS, Liang MH, Newcomer L, et al. Anticardiolipin antibodies and the risk for ischemic stroke and venous thrombosis. *Ann Intern Med*. 1992;117:997-1002.

52. Simioni P, Prandoni P, Lensing AW, et al. The risk of recurrent venous thromboembolism in patients with an arg[506]-gln mutation in the gene for factor V (factor V Leiden). *N Engl J Med*. 1997;336:399-403.

53. Petiti DB, Strom BL, Melmon KL. Duration of warfarin anticoagulant therapy and the probabilities of recurrent thromboembolism and hemorrhage. *Am J Med*. 1986;81:255-259.

54. Schulman S, Svenungsson E, Granqvist S. Anticardiolipin antibodies predict early recurrence of thromboembolism and death among patients with venous thromboembolism following anticoagulant therapy. *Am J Med.* 1998;104:332-338.

55. Rosove MH, Brewer PM. Antiphospholipid thrombosis: clinical course after the first thrombotic event in 70 patients. *Ann Intern Med.* 1992;117:303-308.

56. Khamashta MA, Cuadrado MJ, Mujic F, Taub NA, Hunt BJ, Hughes GR. The management of thrombosis in the antiphospholipid-antibody syndrome. *N Engl J Med.* 1995;332:993-997.

57. Danilenko-Dixon DR, Van Winter JT, Homburger HA. Clinical implications of antiphospholipid antibodies in obstetrics. *Mayo Clin Proc.* 1996;71:1118-1120.

11

12   Acute Coronary Syndromes

Chest pain is a common complaint and is responsible for over 5 million emergency department visits yearly in the United States. Although a majority of individuals do not have cardiac chest pain, nearly 2 million hospital admissions per year are based on a diagnosis of an acute coronary syndrome (ACS); a clinically useful term compatible with myocardial ischemia. It encompasses ST-segment elevation myocardial infarction (MI), non–ST-segment elevation MI, (NSTEMI) and unstable angina, representing a spectrum of atherothrombotic disorders with a common pathobiology.

Pathobiology

The clinical expression of coronary artery disease is driven by a series of pathobiologic events that include plaque disruption and varying degrees of intravascular thromboembolism.[1,2] A majority of patients with unstable angina and NSTEMI have advanced atherosclerotic coronary artery disease with nearly uniform distribution of single-, double-, and triple-vessel involvement; however, it is not the *number* of involved coronary arteries that is unique but the *characteristics* of the underlying atheromatous plaques that are vulnerable to rupture and a dysfunctional endothelium that ineffectively resists thrombosis.[3]

Although plaque disruption is a common theme in ACS, the degree and composition of the associated thrombus burden differ. In contrast to ST-segment elevation MI, the coronary thrombi in patients with unstable angina and NSTEMI are nonocclusive, poorly anchored (ie, prone to embolize), and consist predominantly of platelets with a loose fibrin network[4,5] (Figure 12.1).

Secondary unstable angina or NSTEMI represents a condition wherein myocardial ischemia is provoked by conditions that increase myocardial oxygen demand such as fever, tachycardia, and hypermetabolic states (eg, thyrotoxi-

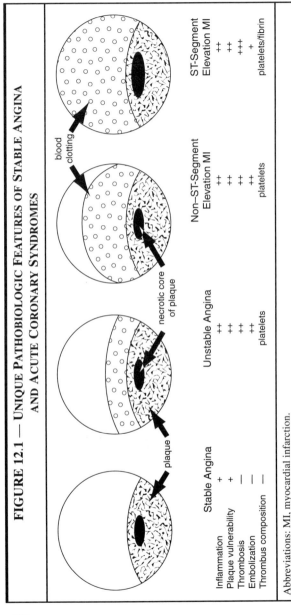

FIGURE 12.1 — UNIQUE PATHOBIOLOGIC FEATURES OF STABLE ANGINA AND ACUTE CORONARY SYNDROMES

	Stable Angina	Unstable Angina	Non–ST-Segment Elevation MI	ST-Segment Elevation MI
Inflammation	+	++	++	++
Plaque vulnerability	+	++	++	++
Thrombosis	—	++	++	+++
Embolization	—	++	++	+
Thrombus composition	—	platelets	platelets	platelets/fibrin

Abbreviations: MI, myocardial infarction.

cosis) as well as by conditions that reduce coronary blood flow (eg, hypotension) or impair oxygen delivery (eg, anemia, hypoxemia).

Patient Characteristics

Although the signs and symptoms that typify ACS vary considerably, a diagnosis is secured for a majority of patients based on the:

- Presence or absence of traditional atherosclerosis risk factors
- Presenting history
- Physical examination
- Electrocardiogram.

Supporting evidence for myocardial necrosis is secured through serial troponin (T or I) or creatine kinase measurements.

Determining the Probability of Coronary Artery Disease

■ Risk Factors

Individuals who have one or more traditional risk factors for atherosclerotic coronary artery disease or who have previously documented disease (prior MI, coronary angiography with one or more vessels containing a stenosis of ≥ 70%, revascularization procedure—prior bypass surgery or PCI) are four to five times more likely to be experiencing myocardial ischemia when they present to the hospital with chest pain than those without existing risk factors or previously documented disease.

■ Electrocardiogram

The surface 12-lead electrocardiogram (ECG) represents an important "first line" diagnostic test in evaluating patients with suspected myocardial ischemia. It is designed to compliment the history and physical examination, providing information that carries considerable predictive value when employed serially in the context of high pretest likelihood of myocardial ischemia (Table 12.1). Although a

TABLE 12.1 — PATIENT CHARACTERISTICS AND ELECTROCARDIOGRAPHIC FEATURES USEFUL IN DETERMINING THE PROBABILITY OF MYOCARDIAL ISCHEMIA

High probability if:
- Known history of myocardial infarction or angina
- Male $\geq$60 or female $\geq$70 years of age
- Variant angina (coronary vasospasm)
- Symmetric T-wave inversion in multiple leads
- ST elevation or depression $\geq$0.5 mm (in 2 or more leads)
- Hypertension, hypercholesterolemia, smoking, family history of coronary artery disease (any combination of these with diabetes mellitus)
- Hemodynamic change or "dynamic" electrocardiographic changes during chest pain

Intermediate probability if:
- Male <60 or female <70 years of age
- History of peripheral vascular disease
- ST segment depression <0.5 mm (in 2 or more leads)
- T-wave inversion $\geq$1 mm in leads with dominant R-waves
- At least 2 positive risk factors (excluding diabetes mellitus)

Low probability if:
- Atypical chest pain
- One risk factor (but *not* diabetes mellitus)
- Normal electrocardiogram (during symptoms)
- Normal physical examination
- T-wave flattening or inversion <1 mm in leads with dominant R wave
- Age <35 years for males or <45 years for females

normal ECG does not fully exclude a diagnosis of unstable angina or NSTEMI, the diagnosis should be questioned when serial tracings performed during symptoms remain normal or unchanged. Nevertheless, if the suspicion for myocardial ischemia remains high, observation, biochemical testing, and additional diagnostic testing should be undertaken (Table 12.2, Figures 12.2, 12.3, and 12.4).[6]

TABLE 12.2 — EARLY EVALUATION STEPS FOR PATIENTS WITH SUSPECTED MYOCARDIAL ISCHEMIA

- The history, physical examination, 12-lead ECG, and initial serum marker tests should be integrated to assign patients with chest pain to 1 of 4 categories: a noncardiac diagnosis, chronic stable angina, possible ACS, and definite ACS.
- Patients with a noncardiac diagnosis should be managed as dictated by the alternative diagnosis.
- Patients with chronic stable angina should be managed according to existing guidelines for the management of patients with chronic stable angina.
- Patients whose symptoms are suggestive of ACS or are felt to be consistent with a definite ACS but whose initial 12-lead ECG and serum cardiac marker levels are normal, should be observed in a facility with cardiac monitoring (eg, chest pain unit) and a repeat ECG and serum marker measurement should be obtained 4 to 8 hours later.
- If the follow-up 12-lead ECG and serum marker measurements are normal, a stress test to provoke ischemia may be performed. Patients with a negative stress test can be managed as outpatients. Patients with a strongly positive stress test are considered to have myocardial ischemia, and in the presence of the clinical picture of acute ischemia, should be admitted to the hospital for further management.
- Patients who are unable to exercise or who have an abnormal resting ECG should have stress myocardial perfusion imaging.
- Patients believed to have an ACS with an abnormal initial 12-lead ECG should be managed based on the findings of the 12-lead ECG. Patients with ST elevation should be evaluated for immediate reperfusion therapy. Patients with new ST depression and/or T-wave abnormalities should be admitted to the hospital for further management.

Abbreviations: ACS, acute coronary syndrome; ECG, electrocardiogram.

ACC/AHA Guidelines for the management of patients with unstable angina and NSTEMI. *Circulation.* 2000;102:1193-1209.

12

FIGURE 12.2 — ST/T-WAVE CHANGES IN PATIENT WITH MYOCARDIAL ISCHEMIA

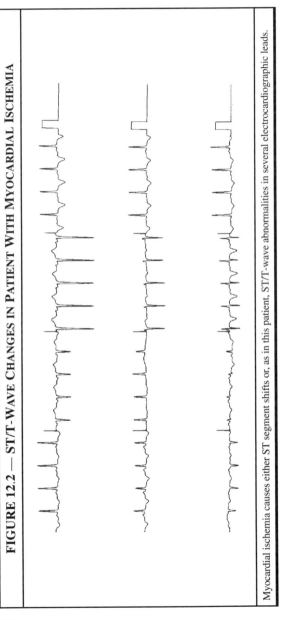

Myocardial ischemia causes either ST segment shifts or, as in this patient, ST/T-wave abnormalities in several electrocardiographic leads.

FIGURE 12.3 — DEEP SYMMETRIC T-WAVE INVERSIONS IN PATIENT WITH MYOCARDIAL ISCHEMIA

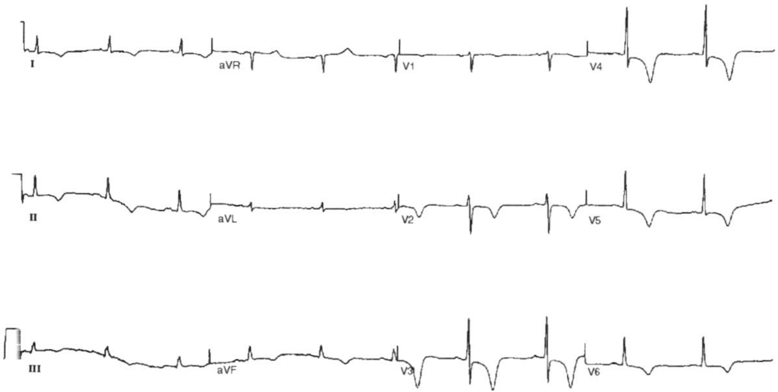

Deep symmetric T-wave inversions in a patient with chest pain at rest and accompanying high-grade stenosis of the proximal left anterior descending coronary artery.

12

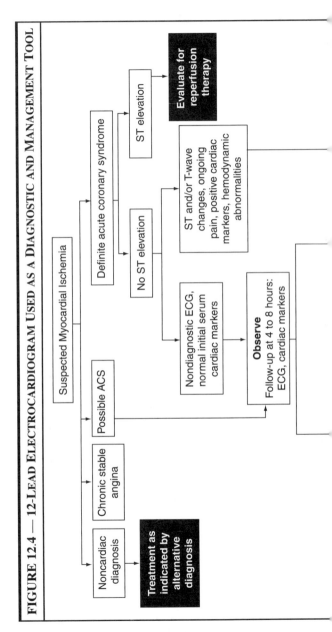

FIGURE 12.4 — 12-LEAD ELECTROCARDIOGRAM USED AS A DIAGNOSTIC AND MANAGEMENT TOOL

Suspected Myocardial Ischemia

Noncardiac diagnosis

Treatment as indicated by alternative diagnosis

Chronic stable angina

Possible ACS

Definite acute coronary syndrome

ST elevation

Evaluate for reperfusion therapy

No ST elevation

ST and/or T-wave changes, ongoing pain, positive cardiac markers, hemodynamic abnormalities

Nondiagnostic ECG, normal initial serum cardiac markers

Observe
Follow-up at 4 to 8 hours: ECG, cardiac markers

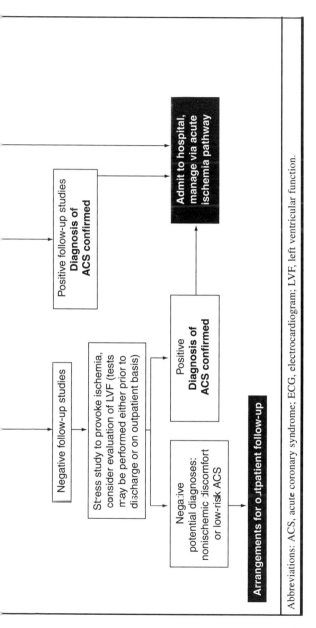

Negative follow-up studies → Stress study to provoke ischemia, consider evaluation of LVF (tests may be performed either prior to discharge or on outpatient basis)

Positive follow-up studies
Diagnosis of ACS confirmed

Positive
Diagnosis of ACS confirmed

Negative potential diagnoses: nonischemic discomfort or low-risk ACS

Arrangements for outpatient follow-up

Admit to hospital, manage via acute ischemia pathway

12

Abbreviations: ACS, acute coronary syndrome; ECG, electrocardiogram; LVF, left ventricular function.

183

- **Classification of Unstable Angina**

The Braunwald Classification System is widely used for evaluating patients with unstable angina.[7] It is comprehensive and has been shown to provide both prognostic information and important insights for management.

- **Risk Stratification**

There are several risk-stratification tools that have been developed over the years; however, the original "high-risk" categorization as defined by the Agency for Health Care Policy and Research[8] provides a clinically useful tool for diagnosis, triage, and management (Table 12.3). The importance of ST-segment shifts[9] and biochemical (cardiac enzyme) abnormalities has been emphasized by several experienced groups.

TABLE 12.3 — HIGH RISK FEATURES IN PATIENTS WITH UNSTABLE ANGINA

High Risk Category (high risk for death or nonfatal myocardial infarction) if *one* or *more* of the following features are present:
- Pulmonary edema with chest pain
- Dynamic mitral insufficiency
- Angina with intermittent S3 gallop or pulmonary rales
- Angina with hypotension
- Prolonged pain (>20 minutes in duration)
- Angina with "dynamic" ST changes
- Persistence of chest pain and electrocardiographic changes despite medical therapy
- Positive troponin T or I assay
- Angina followed by bradyarrhythmias, conduction disturbance or ventricular tachyarrhythmias

---

Hospitalized Patients

- **Monitoring**

All patients admitted to the hospital with suspected myocardial ischemia and a diagnosis of unstable angina or NSTEMI should have 12 to 24 hours of continuous ECG monitoring. When available, ST-segment monitoring should be utilized to aid in the identification of high-risk patients.

■ **Anti-ischemic Therapy**

Optimal management of unstable angina and NSTEMI includes the immediate relief of ischemia and the prevention of serious adverse outcomes (infarction, death). Pharmacologic therapies that address the issue of myocardial ischemia include analgesics, nitrates, β-blockers, and calcium channel blockers. Intra-aortic balloon counterpulsation is a mechanical alternative that should be considered in patients with refractory angina, hemodynamic compromise, or malignant dysarrhythmias associated with myocardial ischemia. In most instances, balloon pumps serve as a bridge to revascularization (Table 12.4).

Antithrombotic Therapy

The pathology of ACS dictates a comprehensive antithrombotic regimen that includes one or more platelet antagonists and an anticoagulant (Tables 12.5 and 12.6).

■ **Platelet Antagonists**

The benefits offered by platelet inhibition are well documented and translate to a 60% to 70% reduction in the likelihood of death or MI. Although aspirin has been the agent used in an overwhelming majority of studies, alternative platelet antagonists, like clopidogrel, should be considered in patients with aspirin allergy, intolerance, or resistance. The advantage a clopidogrel/aspirin combination in ACS was recently confirmed in the Clopidogrel in Unstable Angina to Prevent Recurrent Events (CURE) trial.[10-13]

The intravenous platelet glycoprotein (GP) IIb/IIIa receptor antagonists have added a significant dimension to treatment strategies for ACS. Added benefits (to standard anti-ischemic and antithrombotic therapy) are consistently observed in patients treated medically, as well as in those undergoing percutaneous coronary interventions (PCIs) (Tables 12.5 and 12.6).[14] The greatest overall reduction in adverse events (death, MI, refractory angina) occurs in patients falling within the high-risk category, particularly those with troponin (T or I) positivity.

12

TABLE 12.4 — MEDICAL THERAPY FOR ACUTE CORONARY SYNDROMES

Agent	Indication	Dose	Duration	Alternatives	Comments
ACE inhibitors	ACS	Variable	Variable	—	Greatest benefit in patients with with reduced LVEF and/or clinical heart failure; has antithrombotic properties as well
β-Blockers	ACS	Titrate to heart rate, symptoms	Indefinite	—	—
Calcium channel blockers	ACS	Titrate to symptoms	Variable	—	Used in patients with refractory angina, AF with rapid ventricular response, particularly when β-blocker contraindicated
Lipid-lowering agents	CHD	Variable	Variable	—	Benefit of high-dose statin therapy in early management of ACS
Nitroglycerin	ACS	Titrate to symptoms (IV preferable for rapid titration)	24-48 hours	—	Benefit beyond 48 hours if recurrent ischemia

Abbreviations: ACE, angiotensin-converting enzyme; ACS, acute coronary syndrome; AF, atrial fibrillation; CCB, calcium channel blocker; CHD, coronary heart disease; IV, intravenous; LVEF, left ventricular ejection fraction.

TABLE 12.5 — ANTITHROMBOTIC THERAPY IN ACUTE CORONARY SYNDROMES		
Possible ACS	**High Probability ACS**	**Definite ACS, Refractory Ischemia, and/or High-Risk Features**
Aspirin	Aspirin + LMWH or IV UFH	Aspirin + Clopidogrel + IV UFH* + GPIIb/IIIa antagonist[†]

Abbreviations: ACS, acute coronary syndromes; GP, glycoprotein; IV, intravenous; LMWH, low molecular weight heparin; UFH, unfractionated heparin.

* LMWH may be acceptable alternative or preferred anticoagulant.
† Early angiography/revascularization recommended for high-risk patients.

■ **Anticoagulants**

Intravenous (IV) unfractionated heparin (UFH) given in combination with aspirin is recommended for patients with ACS based on the recognized contribution of platelets and thrombin to arterial thrombosis. Several well-designed studies[15-18] have documented the benefit of UFH with a 30% reduction in the composite outcome of death or MI and an impressive 50% reduction in recurrent/refractory angina.

One of the many recognized challenges of UFH therapy is achieving and maintaining a target level of anticoagulation. Frequent monitoring of the activated partial thromboplastin time (aPTT) is recommended and, when available, point-of-care coagulation instruments (Table 12.7).[19] The duration of treatment is determined by the patient's overall clinical status; however, in most instances, a period of 48 to 72 hours is adequate. Intravenous heparin weaning is recommended to minimize "rebound" thrombin generation.[20]

Low molecular weight heparin (LMWH) represents an attractive treatment alternative and has been shown in several large-scale trials to be superior to aspirin and, at the

TABLE 12.6 — SUMMARY OF ANTITHROMBOTIC THERAPY IN ACUTE CORONARY SYNDROMES

Class/Agent	Dosing	Clinical Indications	Comment
Oral Antiplatelet Therapy			
Aspirin	162-325 mg (initial) 75-160 mg/d (maintenance)	ACS	True aspirin allergy is rare
Clopidogrel (Plavix)	300 mg (loading) 75 mg/d (maintenance)	ACS, PCI-stenting	Combination therapy with aspirin encouraging
Ticlopidine	500 mg (loading) 250 mg bid (maintenance)	PCI-stenting	Adverse effect profile concerning
Intravenous Antiplatelet Therapy			
Abciximab (ReoPro)	0.25 µg/kg bolus, 0.125 µg/kg/min (max 10 µg/min) for 12 to 24 hours	ACS/PCI	Greatest benefit with PCI
Eptifibatide (Integrilin)	180 µg/kg × 2 (10 min apart), 2.0 µg/kg/min for 48 to 72 hours*	ACS/PCI	Double bolus strategy in PCI

Tirofiban (Aggrastat)	0.4 mg/kg/min × 30 min, 0.1 mg/kg/min for 48 to 72 hours*	ACS	Ideal dosing strategy for PCI being investigated
Anticoagulants			
Enoxaparin (Lovenox)	1 mg/kg SC bid*	ACS	Combined use with GPIIb/IIIa antagonist and utilization in PCI being investigated
Dalteparin (Fragmin)	120 IU/kg SC bid* (max 10,000 IU bid)	ACS	Experience with GPIIb/IIIa antagonist and PCI limited
Bivalirudin (Angiomax)	1 mg/kg bolus;* 2.5 mg/kg/h	High-risk PCI, HIT	Investigation of combined therapy with GPIIb/IIIa antagonist ongoing
Lepirudin (Refluden)	0.4 mg/kg bolus,* 0.15 mg/kg/h	HIT	Target aPTT 60-85 sec
Unfractionated heparin	70 U/kg bolus (max 5000 U), 12-15 U/kg/h (max 1000 U/h)	ACS	Target aPTT 60-85 sec, rebound ischemic events following cessation

Abbreviations: ACS, acute coronary syndrome; aPTT, activated partial thromboplastin time; bid, two times per day; GP, glycoprotein; HIT, heparin-induced thrombocytopenia; PCI, percutaneous coronary intervention; SC, subcutaneous.

* Dose adjustment required for renal insufficiency.

12

TABLE 12.7 — PATIENT-SPECIFIC HEPARIN-DOSING NOMOGRAM*			
aPTT	Repeat Bolus[†]	Rate Change[†]	Repeat aPTT
<35 sec	60 U/kg	↑ 4 U/kg/h	4 h
35-49 sec	30 U/kg	↑ 3 U/kg/h	6 h
50-70[‡] sec	0	No change	6 h
71-90 sec	0	↓ 2 U/kg/h	6 h
>90 sec	0	↓ 3 U/kg/h	4 h

Abbreviation: aPTT, activated partial thromboplastin time.

* Initial dose: 60-U/kg bolus (not to exceed 5000 U); maintenance infusion: 15-18 U/kg/h.
† Patients >65 years of age and those receiving fibrinolytics and/or platelet glycoprotein (GP)IIb/IIIa antagonists have reduced heparin requirements.
‡ Target range (for acute coronary syndromes).

very least, equally as efficacious as UFH.[21,22] The findings of two comparative trials, Efficacy and Safety of Subcutaneous Enoxaparin in Non-Q-Wave Coronary Events (ESSENCE)[23] and Thrombolysis in Myocardial Infarction (TIMI) 11B,[24] support LMWH as the standard of care in high-risk patients with ACS. A reduced requirement for coagulation monitoring (with the exception of patients with marked renal insufficiency, ie, creatinine clearance <30 mL/min and those of extremes in body weight <50 kg, >120 kg) coupled with the lower incidence of recurrent refractory ischemia requiring coronary angiography/interventions is responsible for the lower treatment costs for LMWH.

The limitations of UFH during PCI are substantial, not the least of which is its narrow therapeutic index (Figures 12.5 and 12.6).[25]

There are several biologic and practical advantages of LMWH compared with UFH in the management of ACS:

- Rapid subcutaneous absorption
- Predictable pharmacokinetics and pharmacodynamics
- Reduced platelet activation

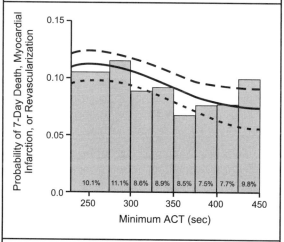

FIGURE 12.5 — NARROW THERAPEUTIC INDEX WITH UNFRACTIONATED HEPARIN IN PERCUTANEOUS CORONARY INTERVENTION

The lowest ischemic event rates are achieved with an activated clotting time (ACT) in excess of 350 seconds.

Chew DP, et al. *Circulation.* 2001;103:961-966.

- Sustained tissue factor pathway inhibitor (TFPI) release
- Reduced heparin-platelet Factor 4–directed antibody production.

■ Low Molecular Weight Heparin in Percutaneous Coronary Intervention

There is emerging evidence in support of LMWH as an alternative to UFH in PCI—an important option in the context of maintaining antithrombotic agent consistency when transitioning from medical to mechanical treatment (Table 12.8). Although the initial experience with enoxaparin in the National Investigators Collaborating on Enoxaparin (NICE)-1 registry employed an intravenous dosing strategy (1.0 mg/kg), there is experience with subcutaneous administration as well.[26] A single center study

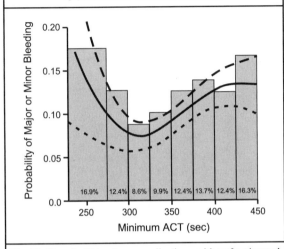

**FIGURE 12.6 — RISK FOR HEMORRHAGE
WITH UNFRACTIONATED HEPARIN
DURING PERCUTANEOUS
CORONARY INTERVENTION**

The likelihood of bleeding complications with unfractionated heparin increases with an activated clotting time (ACT) in excess of 350 seconds.

Chew DP, et al. *Circulation*. 2001;103:961-966.

of 451 patients with unstable angina/NSTEMI performed coronary angioplasty and PCI within 8 hours of a subcutaneous dose (1 mg/kg enoxaparin) (without additional LMWH or UFH). There were no abrupt closures or urgent revascularizations. Preliminary results from the NICE-3 registry suggest that a small additional dose of enoxaparin (0.3 mg/kg IV) could be employed to maintain an adequate level of anticoagulation in cases where the last subcutaneous dose was given 8 or more hours earlier.[27]

- **Combination Pharmacotherapy With
Low Molecular Weight Heparin and
GPIIb/IIIa Receptor Antagonists**
  The combined administration of LMWH and GPIIb/IIIa receptor antagonists is particularly attractive in ACS

given its pathobiology (Figure 12.7) that includes both co-agulation factors (prothrombinase complex) and activated platelets, and their excellent individual track records. The experience to date is encouraging and suggests that it will likely become a widely employed treatment alternative.[28]

■ Direct Thrombin Inhibitors
The direct thrombin inhibitor, hirudin, has shown some promise in preventing early ischemic/thrombotic events[29] in patients with ACS. A related molecule, bivalirudin, offers an advantage over UFH in high-risk coronary angioplasty.[30] Preliminary results with pentasaccharide also look promising.

■ Fibrinolytic Therapy
Fibrinolytic therapy is not beneficial and, in fact, may be detrimental to patients with unstable angina and NSTEMI.[31]

■ Biochemical Markers
Small elevations in biochemical markers of myocyte injury represent an important indicator of plaque activity, thromboembolic potential, and response to treatment. More specifically, an elevated troponin I (or T) in the first 12 hours of an ACS identifies patients at risk for MI and cardiac death[32] and those most likely to benefit from GPIIb/IIIa antagonists and early invasive management.

■ Management Strategies
Patients with unstable angina and NSTEMI, as previously discussed, represent a spectrum of pathobiology and clinical expression of disease. The available information suggests that risk stratification based on the ECG, hemodynamic profile, biochemical (cardiac markers), and in-hospital course is the key to patient-specific management and optimal outcomes (Figure 12.8).

Accumulating data and experience support an early aggressive approach to patient management that includes coronary angiography and revascularization in high-risk individuals (Table 12.9).[33]

193

TABLE 12.8 — CLINICAL EXPERIENCE WITH LMWH ADMINISTERED FOR PCI

Trial/Investigator (No. of Patients)	Route/Dose Administration	GP IIb/IIIa Antagonist	Major Findings
Enoxaparin			
NICE 1 Pilot (60)	IV 1.0 mg/kg	No	Similar safety efficacy and equivalent antifactor Xa to UFH 10,000 U (randomized)
NICE 1 (828)	IV 1.0 mg/kg	No	Favorable bleeding and clinical efficacy. Major non-CABG bleeding 0.5% at 30 days
NICE 4 (818)	IV 0.75 mg/kg	Abciximab	Favorable bleeding and clinical efficacy. Major non-CABG bleeding 0.2% at 30 days
ESSENCE (142)	SC 1.0 mg/kg	No	Major hemorrhage ≤2.0%; similar to UFH
Collet (132)	SC 1.0 mg/kg	No	Antifactor Xa levels maintained for 8 hours post-dose; favorable clinical outcomes
ACUTE 1 (55)	SC 1.0 mg/kg	Tirofiban	Enhanced platelet inhibition by tirofiban (vs UFH; randomized)
ACUTE 2 (525)	SC 1.0 mg/kg	Tirofiban	No difference in bleeding; slight reduction in recurrent ischemia for enoxaparin (vs UFH; randomized)
POLONIA (100)	IC (local delivery)	No	Reduction in neointimal proliferation and late restenosis

Dalteparin			
Kereiakes (107)	IV 40 vs 60 IU/kg	Abciximab	60 IU/kg provided more consistent antithrombotic effect and fewer clinical thrombotic events
Furman/Kereiakes (40)	IV 60 IU/kg	Abciximab	Similar platelet inhibition with abciximab vs UFH 70 U/kg (randomized)
Marmur/DREAM (110)	IV 60-80 IU/kg	Abciximab	Change in the ACT may be used to monitor therapy
Kotani (30)	IC 5000 IU (local delivery)	No	Reduction in neointimal proliferation and late restenosis
Reviparin			
REDUCE (612)	IV 7000 IU + SC to 28 days	No	Similar major bleeding vs UFH (randomized)

Abbreviations: ACT, activated clotting time; CABG, coronary artery bypass graft; DREAM, Diabetes Reduction Approaches with Ramipril and Rosiglitazone Medications; ESSENCE, Efficacy and Safety of Subcutaneous Enoxaparin in Non–Q-Wave Coronary Events); GP, glycoprotein; IC, intracoronary; IV, intravenous; LMWH, low molecular weight heparin; NICE, National Investigators Collaborating on Enoxaparin; PCI, percutaneous coronary intervention; POLONIA, Polish-American Local Lovenox NIR Assessment Study; REDUCE, Reduction of Restenosis After PTCA, Early Administration of Reviparin in a Double-Blind Unfractionated Heparin and Placebo-Controlled Evaluation; SC, subcutaneous; UFH, unfractionated heparin.

Choo JK, et al. *J Thromb Thrombolysis.* 2001. In press.

FIGURE 12.7 — ARTERIAL THROMBOSIS

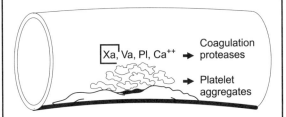

The pivotal roles of platelets and factor Xa in acute arterial thrombosis provide a rationale for combination pharmacotherapy that includes low molecular weight heparin and GPIIb/IIIa receptor antagonists.

Summary

Unstable angina and NSTEMI represent a spectrum of atherothrombotic disorders. Platelet-rich nonocclusive thrombosis and distal embolization are the predominant pathobiologic features that develop on a background of advanced atherosclerosis. Anti-ischemic and antithrombotic therapy, including aspirin, heparin, and IV GPIIb/IIIa receptor antagonists, are the cornerstones of treatment. An aggressive approach to diagnosis and management is favored in high-risk patients with hemodynamic instability, recurrent/refractory ischemia, and biochemical markers reflecting myocyte damage.

REFERENCES

1. Falk E. Unstable angina with fatal outcome: dynamic coronary thrombosis leading to infarction and/or sudden death. Autopsy evidence of recurrent mural thormbosis with peripheral embolization culminating in total vascular occlusion. *Circulation.* 1985;71:699-708.

2. Davies MJ, Thomas A. Thrombosis and acute coronary-artery lesions in sudden cardiac ischemic death. *N Engl J Med.* 1984;310:1137-1140.

3. Furchgott RF, Zawadzki JV. The obligatory role of endothelial cells in the relaxation of arterial smooth muscle by acetylcholine. *Nature.* 1980;288:373-376.

4. Sherman CT, Litvack F, Grundfest W, et al. Coronary angioscopy in patients with unstable angina pectoris. *N Engl J Med*. 1986;315:913-919.

5. Kragel AH, Gertz SD, Roberts WC. Morphologic comparison of frequency and types of acute lesions in the major epicardial coronary arteries in unstable angina pectoris, sudden coronary death and acute myocardial infarction. *J Am Coll Cardiol*. 1991;18:801-808.

6. Braunwald E, Antman EM, Beasley JW, et al. ACC/AHA guidelines for the management of patients with unstable angina and non–ST-segment elevation myocardial infarction: executive summary and recommendations. A report of the American College of Cardiology/American Heart Association task force on practice guidelines (committee on the management of patients with unstable angina). *Circulation*. 2000;102:1193-1209.

7. Braunwald E. Unstable angina. A classification. *Circulation*. 1989:80:410-414.

8. Braunwald E, Mark DB, Jones RH, et al. Unstable angina: diagnosis and management. Clinical Practice Guideline Number 10. Agency for Health Care Policy and Research and the National Heart, Lung, and Blood Institute, Public Health Service, US Department of Health and Human Services, Rockville, MD, 1994.

9. Kaul P, Fu Y, Chang WC, et al. Prognostic value of ST-segment depression in acute coronary syndromes: insights from PARAGON-A applied to GUSTO-IIb. *J Am Coll Cardiol*. 2001;38:64-71.

10. Ryan TJ, Anderson JL, Antman EM, et al. ACC/AHA guidelines for the management of patients with acute myocardial infarction: a report of the American College of Cardiology/American Heart Association Task Force on Practice Guidelines (Committee on Management of Acute Myocardial Infarction). *J Am Coll Cardiol*. 1996;28:1328-1428.

11. Ryan TJ, Antman EM, Brooks NH, et al, for the Committee of Management of Acute Myocardial Infarction. 1999 Update: ACC/AHA guidelines for the management of patients with acute myocardial infarction. A report of the American College Cardiology/American Heart Association Task Force on Practice Guidelines. *J Am Coll Cardiol*. 1999;34:890-911.

12. CAPRIE Steering Committee. A randomised, blinded, trial of clopidogrel versus aspirin in patients at risk of ischaemic events (CAPRIE). *Lancet*. 1996;348:1329-1339.

13. The CURE Investigators. Effects of clopidogrel in addition to aspirin in patients with acute coronary syndromes without ST-segment elevation. *N Engl J Med*. 2001;345:494-502.

12

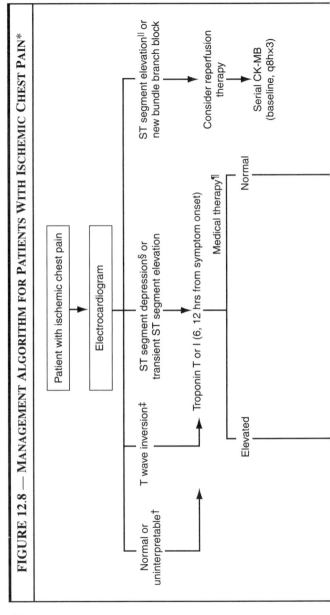

FIGURE 12.8 — MANAGEMENT ALGORITHM FOR PATIENTS WITH ISCHEMIC CHEST PAIN*

Patient with ischemic chest pain

Electrocardiogram

Normal or uninterpretable†

T wave inversion‡

ST segment depression§ or transient ST segment elevation

ST segment elevation‖ or new bundle branch block

Troponin T or I (6, 12 hrs from symptom onset)

Elevated

Normal

Medical therapy¶

Consider reperfusion therapy

Serial CK-MB (baseline, q8h×3)

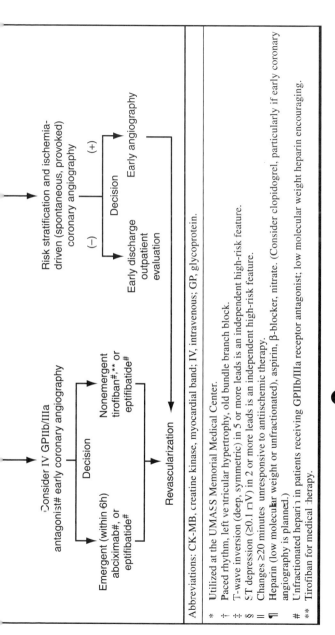

Consider IV GPIIb/IIIa antagonist# early coronary angiography

Decision

Emergent (within 6h) abciximab#, or eptifibatide#

Nonemergent tirofiban#,** or eptifibatide#

Revascularization

Risk stratification and ischemia-driven (spontaneous, provoked) coronary angiography

Decision

(−) Early discharge outpatient evaluation

(+) Early angiography

Abbreviations: CK-MB, creatine kinase, myocardial band; IV, intravenous; GP, glycoprotein.

* Utilized at the UMASS Memorial Medical Center.
† Paced rhythm, left ventricular hypertrophy, old bundle branch block.
‡ T-wave inversion (deep, symmetric) in 5 or more leads is an independent high-risk feature.
§ ST depression (≥0.1 mV) in 2 or more leads is an independent high-risk feature.
‖ Changes ≥20 minutes unresponsive to antiischemic therapy.
¶ Heparin (low molecular weight or unfractionated), aspirin, β-blocker, nitrate. (Consider clopidogrel, particularly if early coronary angiography is planned.)
# Unfractionated heparin in patients receiving GPIIb/IIIa receptor antagonist; low molecular weight heparin encouraging.
** Tirofiban for medical therapy.

TABLE 12.9 — REVASCULARIZATION IN ACUTE CORONARY SYNDROMES WITHOUT ST-SEGMENT ELEVATION

Coronary Angiography	Mode of Treatment
Left main disease (≥50% stenosis)	
Surgical candidate	CABG
Nonsurgical candidate	PCI
3-Vessel disease, LVEF <50%	CABG
Multivessel disease, LVEF ≥50%, (nondiabetic)	PCI
1- or 2-Vessel disease, large areas of reversible ischemia	CABG or PCI
2-Vessel disease, including proximal LAD, LVEF <50%	CABG
Proximal LAD disease	PCI or CABG

Abbreviations: CABG, coronary artery bypass grafting; LAD, left anterior descending coronary artery; LVEF, left ventricular ejection fraction; PCI, percutaneous coronary intervention.

14. Kong DF, Califf RM, Miller DP, et al. Clinical outcomes of therapeutic agents that block the platelet glycoprotein IIb/IIIa integrin in ischemic heart disease. *Circulation*. 1998;98:2829-2835.

15. Theroux P, Ouimet H, McCans J, et al. Aspirin, heparin, or both to treat acute unstable angina. *N Engl J Med*. 1988;319:1105-1111.

16. Cohen M, Adams PC, Hawkins L, Bach M, Fuster V. Usefulness of antithrombotic therapy in resting angina pectoris or non-Q-wave myocardial infarction in preventing death and myocardial infarction (a pilot study from the Antithrombotic Therapy in Acute Coronary Syndromes Study Group). *Am J Cardiol*. 1990;66:1287-1292.

17. The RISC Group. Risk of myocardial infarction and death during treatment with low dose aspirin and intravenous heparin in men with unstable coronary artery disease. *Lancet*. 1990;336:827-830.

18. Cohen M, Adams PC, Parry G, et al. Combination antithrombotic therapy in unstable rest angina and non-Q-wave infarction in nonprior aspirin users. Primary end points analysis from the ATACS trial. Antithrombotic Therapy in Acute Coronary Syndromes Research Group. *Circulation*. 1994;89:81-88.

19. Becker RC, Ball SP, Eisenberg P, et al. A randomized, multicenter trial of weight-adjusted intravenous heparin dose titration and point-of-care coagulation monitoring in hospitalized patients with active thromboembolic disease. Antithrombotic Therapy Consortium Investigators. *Am Heart J.* 1999;137:59-71.

20. Becker RC, Spencer FA, Li Y, et al. Thrombin generation after the abrupt cessation of intravenous unfractionated heparin among patients with acute coronary syndromes: potential mechanisms for heightened prothrombotic potential. *J Am Coll Cardiol.* 1999;34:1020-1027.

21. Gurfinkel EP, Manos EJ, Mejail RI, et al. Low molecular weight heparin versus regular heparin or aspirin in the treatment of unstable angina and silent ischemia. *J Am Coll Cardiol.* 1995;26:313-318.

22. Fragmin and Fast Revascularisation During Instability in Coronary Artery Disease (FRISC II) Investigators. Long-term low-molecular-mass heparin in unstable coronary artery disease: FRISC II prospective randomised multicentre study. *Lancet.* 1999;354:701-707.

23. Cohen M, Demers C, Gurfinkel EP, et al. A comparison of low-molecular-weight heparin with unfractionated heparin for unstable coronary artery disease. Efficacy and Safety of Subcutaneous enoxaparin in Non-Q-Wave Coronary Events Study Group. *N Engl J Med.* 1997;337:447-452.

24. Antman EM, McCabe CH, Gurfinkel EP, et al. Enoxaparin prevents death and cardiac ischaemic events in unstable angina/non-Q-wave myocardial infarction. Results of the Thrombolysis in Myocardial Infarction (TIMI) 11B trial. *Circulation.* 1999;100:1593-1601.

25. Choo JK, Kereiakas DJ. Low molecular weight heparin therapy for percutaneous coronary intervention: a practice in evolution. *J Thromb Thrombolysis.* 2001. In press.

26. Collet JP, Montalescot G, Lison L, et al. Percutaneous coronary intervention after subcutaneous enoxaparin pretreatment in patients with unstable angina pectoris. *Circulation.* 2001;103:658-663.

27. Ferguson JJ. Special report from the 22nd Congress of the European Society of Cardiology. Amsterdam, The Netherlands. August, 2000.

28. Kereiakas DJ, Grines C, Fry E, et al for the NICE-1 and NICE 4 Investigators. Enoxaparin and abciximab adjunctive pharmacotherapy during percutaneous coronary intervention. *J Invasive Cardiol.* 2001; 13:272-278.

29. The Global Use of Strategies to Open Occluded Coronary Arteries (GUSTO) IIB Investigators. A comparison of recombinant hirudin with heparin for the treatment of acute coronary syndromes. *N Engl J Med.* 1996;335:775-782.

30. Bittl JA, Strony J, Brinker JA, et al. Treatment with bivalirudin (hirulog) as compared with heparin during coronary angioplasty for unstable or postinfarction angina. Hirulog Angioplasty Study Investigators. *N Engl J Med*. 1995;333:764-769.

31. The Thrombolysis in Myocardial Ischemia (TIMI)-IIIB Investigators. Effects of tissue plasminogen activator and a comparison of early invasive and conservative strategies in unstable angina and non-Q-wave myocardial infarction. Results of TIMI IIIB Trial. *Circulation*. 1994;89:1545-1556.

32. Antman EM, Tanasijevic MJ, Thompson B, et al. Cardiac-specific troponin I levels to predict the risk of mortality in patients with acute coronary syndromes. *N Engl J Med*. 1996;335:1342-1349.

33. Smith SC, Dove JT, Jacobs AK, et al. ACC/AHA guidelines of percutaneous coronary intervention (revision of the 1993 PTCA guidelines)—executive summary. A report of the Amreican College of Cardiology/American Heart Association Task Force on Practice Guidelines (committee to revise the 1993 guidelines for percutaneous transluminal coronary angioplasty). *J Am Coll Cardiol*. 2001;37:2215-2238.

13   Acute Myocardial Infarction

Rupture of an atherosclerotic plaque with subsequent thrombosis due to platelet aggregation and activation of the intrinsic and extrinsic pathways of coagulation is the initiating event in patients with acute coronary syndromes (ACS). When the developing thrombus causes complete occlusion and cessation of blood flow, an acute myocardial infarction (AMI) ensues, heralded by ST-segment elevation on the electrocardiogram (ECG).

The initial goals of antithrombotic and fibrinolytic therapy in patients with ST-segment elevation MI are to achieve rapid and sustained patency of the infarct-related artery and physiologic myocardial perfusion through a combination of pharmacologic agents that:

- Inhibit platelet aggregation
- Inhibit thrombin generation and activity
- Activate endogenous pathways of fibrinolysis, either alone or as an adjunct to mechanical reperfusion modalities.

The long-term goals are to prevent:

- Coronary artery reocclusion
- Thrombotic sequelae of new plaque rupture
- Formation and subsequent embolization of mural thrombi.

Antiplatelet Agents

The most compelling evidence for aspirin's benefit in acute MI emerged from the Second International Study of Infarct Survival (ISIS-2)[3] that evaluated outcomes in 17,187 AMI patients treated with intravenous (IV) streptokinase (SK), 160 mg of oral aspirin, both, or neither. Aspirin alone was associated with a 35-day mortality reduction of 23% that increased to 42% when combined with SK (Figure 13.1). In addition, aspirin reduced the risk of nonfatal reinfarction by 49% and nonfatal stroke by 46%. Aspirin re-

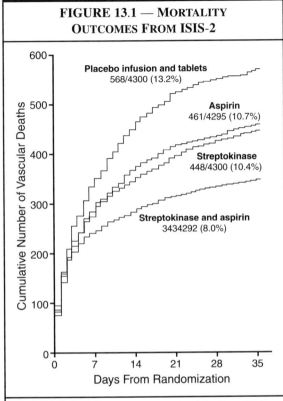

FIGURE 13.1 — MORTALITY OUTCOMES FROM ISIS-2

Placebo infusion and tablets
568/4300 (13.2%)

Aspirin
461/4295 (10.7%)

Streptokinase
448/4300 (10.4%)

Streptokinase and aspirin
3434292 (8.0%)

Cumulative Number of Vascular Deaths

Days From Randomization

Abbreviation: ISIS-2, Second International Studies of Infarct Survival.

ISIS-2. *Lancet.* 1988;11:349-360.

duced the rate of early reinfarction due to SK-induced platelet activation (3.8% vs 1.3%).[1] The absolute number of lives saved with aspirin increases dramatically with advancing age: 2.5 per 100 patients treated <60 years of age, 7 to 8 per 100 treated >60 years of age.

Thus, a dose of 160 mg to 325 mg of nonenteric-coated aspirin represents the cornerstone of initial antiplatelet therapy in patients with AMI. Alternatively, aspirin can be administered as a 325-mg suppository in patients with severe nausea or vomiting. Aspirin is contraindicated in patients with a hypersensitivity to salicylates and should be used with caution in patients with active peptic ulcer disease.[4]

The benefits of aspirin are seen regardless of patient age or gender and across the broad spectrum of patients with ACS, cerebrovascular disease, and chronic atherosclerotic disease. Lifelong therapy is recommended, at a dose ranging from 80 to 325 mg/day.[1]

Given the rapid onset of platelet inhibition derived from a 300-mg dose of clopidogrel (four 75-mg tablets) and its benefit compared with aspirin in the Clopidogrel vs Aspirin in Patients at Risk for Ischemic Events (CAPRIE) study, clopidogrel is considered an acceptable alternative for patients unable to take aspirin.[5] The favorable results reported in the Clopidogrel in Unstable Angina to Prevent Recurrent Ischemic Events (CURE) trial, where the combination of clopidogrel and aspirin reduced the cumulative incidence of death, myocardial infarction, and stroke by 20%, at the cost of a slightly higher risk of non–life-threatening bleeding, support combined pharmacotherapy in patients with acute coronary syndromes.[39]

Fibrinolytic Therapy

The observations of DeWood and other investigators[2,4] that thrombotic occlusion of a coronary artery is the most common cause of acute ST-elevation infarction led to the development of plasminogen activators (summarized in Chapter 4, *Fibrinolytic Agents*). All of the available fibrinolytic agents activate single-chain plasma plasminogen via a direct or indirect enzymatic reaction to the active fibrinolytic agent, double-chain plasmin.[6] Characteristics of the currently available agents, SK, anistreplase, recombinant tissue plasminogen activator (rtPA), reteplase (rPA), and tenecteplase (TNK-tPA) are shown in Table 13.1.[4]

■ Benefits of Fibrinolytic Therapy

Observations from experimental animal models and clinical studies performed in humans demonstrated that prompt recanalization of the infarct artery salvaged myocardium, preserved left ventricular performance, and im-

TABLE 13.1 — COMPARISON OF APPROVED FIBRINOLYTIC AGENTS

Feature of Agent	Streptokinase	Anistreplase	Alteplase	Reteplase	Tenecteplase
Dose	1.5 MU in 30-60 min	30 mg in 5 min	100 mg in 90 min	10 U × 2 over 30 min	0.55 mg/kg over 5-10 sec
Bolus administration	No	Yes	No	Yes	Yes
Antigenic	Yes	Yes	No	No	No
Allergic reactions (hypotension most common)	Yes	Yes	No	No	No
Systemic fibrinogen depletion	Marked	Marked	Mild	Moderate	Mild
90-min patency rates (%)	~50	~65	~75	~75	~75
TIMI grade 3 flow (%)	32	43	54	60	~60
Mortality rate in most recent comparative trials (%)	7.3	10.5	7.2	6.0	6.0
Cost per dose (USD)	$294	$2200	$2200	$2200	$2200

Abbreviations: TIMI, Thrombolysis in Myocardial Infarction; USD, United States dollars.

From: ACC/AHA Joint Guideline Statement.

proved outcome in a time-dependent fashion.[11,12] Treatment administered within the initial 2 hours provides the greatest overall benefit.[6] A meta-analysis including all placebo-controlled trials of fibrinolytic therapy[7] that randomized 1000 or more patients with suspected MI demonstrated an 18% reduction in 30-day mortality. The largest of these trials, ISIS-2,[3] demonstrated an additive benefit of aspirin, which was associated with a mortality reduction of 53% when given in combination with SK within 4 hours of symptoms. Survival benefit was evident across a broad range of subgroups, including:

- Patients with ST elevation or left bundle branch block (LBBB) within 12 hours of symptom onset
- Diabetics
- Advanced age
- Prior MI
- Systolic blood pressure considered either low (<100 mm Hg) or high.

Although the magnitude of benefit from fibrinolytic therapy is maximal within the first "golden hour,"[13] the window of opportunity extends to 12 hours or more (in select cases) from symptom onset.[3,8,9]

■ **Comparative Trials**

Several randomized clinical trials have compared the most widely used fibrinolytic agents, SK and tissue plasminogen activator (tPA): Gruppo Italiano per lo Studio della Sopravvivenza nell'Infarto Miocardico (GISSI)-2[10], ISIS-3[11], and Global Utilization of SK and tPA for Occluded Coronary Arteries (GUSTO)-1[12] (Table 13.2). The largest trial, GUSTO-1, randomized 41,000 patients with ST-segment elevation to one of four treatment strategies. Accelerated "front-loaded" tPA with IV unfractionated heparin reduced 30-day mortality by 15% compared with SK with IV or subcutaneous unfractionated heparin (Figure 13.2). This benefit was maintained at 1 year (Figure 13.2) although hemorrhagic stroke occurred more often with tPA (0.7%) than with SK (0.4%), a net clinical benefit was still achieved with tPA, as evidenced by nine fewer deaths or disabling strokes per 1000 patients treated.[12] Other complications of MI occurred less frequently as well, including heart fail-

TABLE 13.2 — MORTALITY OUTCOME IN COMPARATIVE TRIALS OF FIBRINOLYTIC THERAPY

Study	No. of Patients	Agents, Dose	Time (h)	Follow-up	Mortality			
					Therapy (%)	Control (%)	RRR (%)/ ARR (%)	P Value
GISSI-2	12,490	SK 1.5 MU, 0.5-1 h vs tPA 100 mg, 3 h; heparin SQ vs control	< 6	Hospital	SK, 8.6	tPA, 9.0	—	Not significant
International Study Group	20,891	SK 1.5 MU, 0.5-1 h vs tPA 100 mg, 3 h; heparin SQ vs control	< 6	Hospital	SK, 8.5	tPA, 8.9	—	Not significant
ISIS-3	41,291	SK 1.5 MU, 1 h, APSAC 30 U, 3-5 min, duteplase 0.6 MU/kg; heparin SQ vs control	< 24	35 d	SK, 10.5	APSAC, 10.6; tPA, 10.3	—	Not significant
INJECT	6,010	SK 1.5 MU, 1 h, rPA 10 U, repeated after 30 min; heparin IV to all	< 12	35 d	SK, 9.53	rPA, 9.02	0.51	Not significant

GUSTO-1	41,02_	SK 1.5 MU, 1 h + heparin SQ or IV or SK 1.0 MU 1 h + tPA 1.0 mg/kg 1 h + heparin, or tPA up to 100 mg 1.5 h + heparin	< 6	30 d	SK-SQ heparin, 7.2; SK-IV heparin, 7.4	SK, 7.0; tPA, 6.3; rtPA, 6.3	Accelerated tPA vs SK 14/1.0	0.001
GUSTO-III	15,059	tPA up to 100 mg, 1.5 h or rPA 10 U, repeated after 30 min; heparin IV to all	< 6	30 d	tPA, 7.24	rPA, 7.47	0.23	0.54
COBALT	7,169	tPA up to 100 mg, 1.5 h rtPA 50-mg bolus, repeated (50 or 40 mg) after 30 min; heparin IV to all	< 6	30 d	tPA accelerated, 7.53	tPA 2 bolus, 7.98	0.45	Not significant

Abbreviations: APSAC, anisoylated plasminogen-streptokinase activator complex; ARR, absolute risk reduction; COBALT, Continuous Infusion versus Double-Bolus Administration of Alteplase; GISSI, Grupo Italiano per lo Studio della Sopravvivenza neu'Infarcto Miocardico; GUSTO, Global Use of Strategies to Open Occluded Coronary Arteries; INJECT, International Joint Efficacy Comparison of Thrombolytics; ISIS, International Study of Infarct Survival; IV, intravenous; MU, megaunit; rPA, reteplase; RRR, relative risk reduction; rtPA, recombinant tissue plasminogen activator; SK, streptokinase; SQ, subcutaneous; tPA, tissue plasminogen activator; U, unit.

Cairns JA, et al. *Chest.* 1998;114(suppl);636S.

13

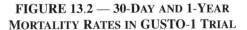

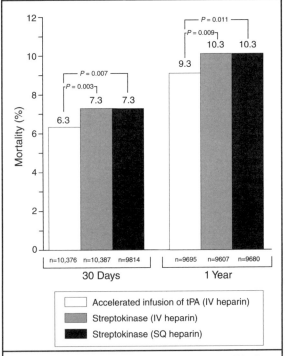

FIGURE 13.2 — 30-DAY AND 1-YEAR MORTALITY RATES IN GUSTO-1 TRIAL

Abbreviations: IV, intravenous; SQ, subcutaneous; tPA, tissue plasminogen activator.

Superior outcome occurred in the treatment group receiving front-loaded tPA and IV heparin.

ure, cardiogenic shock, allergic reactions, and arrhythmias. The GUSTO angiographic substudy provided strong evidence that rapid achievement of Thrombolysis in Myocardial Infarction (TIMI) 3 (physiologic) flow within the infarct-related coronary artery was a key determinant of favorable outcomes.[13,14] TIMI-3 flow rates at 90 minutes in tPA-treated patients were 55%, compared with an average of 29% in SK-treated patients. Irrespective of the fibrinolytic agent, mortality was lowest (4.2%) in patients with

TIMI-3 flow and highest (8.2%) in patients with TIMI 0 or 1 flow at 90 minutes.[14]

In addition to overall survival, TIMI-3 flow status correlated closely with global and infarct region left ventricular function and cavity dilation. These data provided a "proof of concept" platform for fibrinolytic therapy and an evidence-based rationale for establishing early and complete coronary arterial patency and myocardial perfusion as the primary goals of treatment.[4,15-17]

Reteplase, a deletion mutant of tPA, and TNK-tPA, a single-bolus mutant of tPA, were both found to be similar in outcome and efficacy compared with tPA in the GUSTO-3[15] and Assessment of the Safety and Efficacy of a New Thrombolytic (ASSENT)-II[16] trials.

Complications of Fibrinolytic and Adjunctive Therapy

The major complication associated with fibrinolytic therapy is bleeding, with intracranial hemorrhage representing the most feared and devastating event. The risk of intracranial bleeding ranges from 0.3% in low-risk patients (<65 years of age) to 5% in patients >75 years old with additional risk factors. Nearly two thirds of patients with intracranial hemorrhage will die or sustain significant neurologic disability, particularly in patients >75 years of age, in whom the case fatality rate exceeds 90%.[18] Other sites of serious bleeding, such as genitourinary, gastrointestinal, or retroperitoneal, are uncommon (<5%) but can be life-threatening if not quickly recognized and treated. The Fibrinolytic Therapy Trialists reported that for each 1,000 patients treated with a fibrinolytic agent, seven major noncerebral hemorrhages and two nonfatal strokes would result, while preventing 18 deaths over 35 days following the MI.[7,19] The incidence of access-site hemorrhage is decreasing with the use of smaller-bore catheters and lower doses of heparin. Allergic reactions occur commonly (1% to 5%) with SK, but true anaphylactic reactions are rare (<0.5%). Hypotension ranges from 5% to 7% with SK and is less common (2% to 4%) with tPA. Reinfarction rates range from 2% to 4%, depending on the use of conjunctive heparin and aspirin.[19] Table 13.3 provides a current sum-

TABLE 13.3 — CONTRAINDICATIONS AND CAUTIONS FOR USE OF FIBRINOLYTIC AGENTS IN MYOCARDIAL INFARCTION*

Contraindications
- Previous hemorrhagic stroke at any time; other strokes or cerebrovascular events within 1 year
- Known intracranial neoplasm
- Active internal bleeding (does not include menses)
- Suspected aortic dissection

Cautions/Relative Contraindications
- Severe uncontrolled hypertension on presentation (blood pressure >180/110 mm Hg)†
- History of prior cerebrovascular accident or known intracerebral pathology not covered in contraindications
- Current use of anticoagulants in therapeutic doses (INR 2 to 3); known bleeding diathesis
- Recent trauma (within 2 to 4 weeks), including head trauma or traumatic or prolonged (>10 min) CPR or major surgery (<3 weeks)
- Noncompressible vascular punctures
- Recent (within 2 to 4 weeks) internal bleeding
- For streptokinase/anistreplase: prior exposure (especially within 5 d to 2 y) or prior allergic reaction
- Pregnancy
- Active peptic ulcer
- History of chronic severe hypertension

Abbreviations: CPR, cardiopulmonary resuscitation; INR, international normalized ratio.

* Viewed as advisory for clinical decision making and may not be all inclusive or definitive.
† Could be an absolute contraindication in low-risk patients with myocardial infarction.

From: ACC/AHA Joint Guideline Statement.

mary of contraindications and cautions for the administration of fibrinolytic agents.

A novel strategy, employing a reduced 50-mg bolus dose of tPA, followed by immediate angiography and "facilitated" per cutaneous coronary intervention (PCI) for TIMI grade 0, 1, or 2 flow, provided encouraging results.[20] One of the great challenges faced by clinicians is the determination of successful coronary fibrinolysis and physiologic myocardial perfusion. If the patient develops sudden and significant relief of chest pain, full resolution of ST elevation on the ECG, and experiences concomitant salvos of an accelerated idioventricular rhythm, patency and reperfusion are more likely; however, this triad is seen in <10% of patients.[21] Accordingly, mounting interest has focused on rapid resolution of ST elevation determined by continuous (automated) ST-segment analysis as a means to establish a diagnosis.

Recommendations for the Use of Fibrinolytic Agents

The indications for fibrinolytic therapy are summarized in the 1999 AHA/ACC consensus guidelines for AMI[4] (Table 13.4). Patients <75 years of age with ischemic chest pain and ST elevation greater than 0.1 mV in two or more contiguous leads or bundle branch block presenting within 12 hours of symptom onset are considered optimal candidates.[4] In patients >75 years of age, the absolute benefit of therapy is substantial, although the relative benefit is somewhat less than in patients <75.[7] Benefit also diminishes for treatment given within 12 to 24 hours of symptoms, as well as in patients with blood pressure >180/110 mm Hg, due to the increased risk of intracranial hemorrhage.

Despite the strong clinical trial data supporting these recommendations, a substantial number of patients (25% or more) identified as ideal candidates (based on existing criteria) remain untreated, particularly those at highest risk, such as patients with LBBB or heart failure.[22] Thus further efforts are needed to ensure that patients who could benefit from an established and potentially lifesaving means of therapy receive it in a timely manner.

13

TABLE 13.4 — DIAGNOSTIC AND TREATMENT MEASURES IN PATIENTS WITH ST ELEVATION OR BUNDLE BRANCH BLOCK

Initial Diagnostic Measures
- Use continuous ECG, automated BP, HR monitoring
- Take targeted history (for AMI inclusions, thrombolysis exclusions), check vital signs, perform focused examination
- Start IV(s), draw blood for serum cardiac markers, hematology, chemistry, lipid profile
- Obtain 12-lead ECG
- Obtain chest x-ray (preferably upright)

General Treatment Measures
- Aspirin, 160-325 mg (chew and swallow)
- Nitroglycerin, sublingual: test for Prinzmetal's angina, reversible spasm; anti-ischemic, antihypertensive effects
- Oxygen: sparse data; probably indicated, first 2 to 3 h in all; continue if arterial oxygen saturation is low (<90%)
- Adequate analgesia: small doses of morphine (2 to 4 mg) as needed

Specific Treatment Measures
- Reperfusion therapy: goal—door-to-needle time <30 min; door-to-dilatation time <60 min
- Conjunctive antithrombotics: aspirin, heparin (especially with tPA, rPA, or TNKase)
- Adjunctive therapies: Beta-adrenoceptor blockade if eligible, intravenous nitroglycerin (for anti-ischemic or antihypertensive effects), ACE inhibitor (especially with large or anterior AMI, heart failure without hypotension [SBP >100 mm Hg], previous MI)
- Early use of statins

Abbreviations: ACE, angiotensin converting enzyme; AMI, acute myocardial infarction; BP, blood pressure; ECG, electrocardiogram; HR, heart rate; IVs, intravenous administrations; rPA, retaplase; SBP, systolic blood pressure; TNKase, tenectaplase; tPA, tissue plasminogen activator.

From: ACC/AHA Joint Guideline Statement.

Primary Percutaneous Coronary Intervention

Although fibrinolytic therapy can be administered in virtually any hospital with minimal delay, the rate of TIMI-3 flow plateaus at approximately 50% to 60%. Mechanical reperfusion, using balloon angioplasty or primary coronary stenting, can attain TIMI-3 flow in >85% of patients. A pooled analysis of 10 randomized trials of PCI and fibrinolytic therapy performed by Weaver[23] demonstrated significantly lower rates of the following in favor of mechanical intervention:

- Death (4.4% vs 6.5%)
- Nonfatal reinfarction (7.2% vs 11.9%)
- Hemorrhagic stroke (0.1% vs 1.1%).

A portion of the early benefits had diminished by 1 year.[24,25]

The benefit derived from primary PCI, as with fibrinolytic therapy, is time dependent. Delays beyond 90 minutes from hospital arrival are not uncommon in clinical practice.[26] In addition, only about 20% of US hospitals have onsite capabilities and of those one quarter are capable of mobilizing a catheterization team within 60 minutes. Thus for primary PCI to achieve maximal benefit, it must be initiated in a timely manner (60 to 90 minutes of hospital arrival) within 12 hours of symptom onset (or beyond 12 hours if ischemic symptoms persist) by persons skilled in the procedure and supported by an experienced catheterization laboratory team. Patients with cardiogenic shock[27] as well as those who are not candidates for fibrinolytic therapy should be considered for immediate coronary angiography and primary PCI.[4]

Overcoming Thrombolytic Resistance

With currently used fibrinolytic strategies, vessel patency (TIMI-2 or 3 flow) is achieved in approximately 60% to 85% of patients, but physiologic reperfusion (TIMI-3 flow), is restored in barely 50%. This "resistance" to optimal reperfusion may be driven by several mechanisms (Figure 13.3).[28-30]

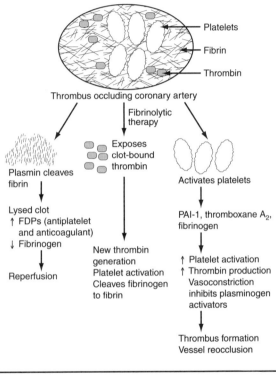

FIGURE 13.3 — THROMBOLYTIC RESISTANCE DUE TO ACTIVATION OF THROMBIN AND PLATELETS

Platelets

Fibrin

Thrombin

Thrombus occluding coronary artery

Fibrinolytic therapy

Exposes clot-bound thrombin

Plasmin cleaves fibrin

Activates platelets

Lysed clot
↑ FDPs (antiplatelet and anticoagulant)
↓ Fibrinogen

PAI-1, thromboxane A$_2$, fibrinogen

Reperfusion

New thrombin generation
Platelet activation
Cleaves fibrinogen to fibrin

↑ Platelet activation
↑ Thrombin production
Vasoconstriction inhibits plasminogen activators

Thrombus formation
Vessel reocclusion

Abbreviations: FDP, fibrin/fibrinogen degradation product; PAI-1, plasminogen activator inhibitor-1.

Moliterno DJ, Topol EJ. *Thromb Haemost.* 1997;78:214-219.

The most commonly used antithrombotic strategy, unfractionated heparin (UFH), does not inhibit clot-bound thrombin. The traditional antiplatelet agent, aspirin, has been shown to decrease the risk of reocclusion and reinfarction[3] following coronary thrombolysis but does not inhibit activation of glycoprotein (GP)IIb/IIIa receptors (and fibrinogen-mediated platelet aggregation).

Several trials have examined the safety and efficacy of combination pharmacotherapy employing fibrinolytic agents and GPIIb/IIIa receptor antagonists. The Integrelin and Reduced Dose of Thrombolytics in Acute Myocardial Infarction (INTRO-AMI) trial evaluated the combination of eptifibatide and reduced-dose tPA, demonstrating a rate of TIMI-3 flow approaching 75% at 90 minutes.[31] The TIMI-14 study tested the combination of abciximab and either reduced dose tPA, rPA, or SK.[32] Abciximab alone produced a TIMI-3 flow rate of 32% at 90 minutes, similar to that obtained with SK alone. The combination of abciximab and SK produced only modest improvement in TIMI flow grade, with a significant increase in hemorrhage. The combination of half-dose tPA (15 mg bolus plus 35 mg over 60 minutes) and abciximab produced TIMI-3 flow rates of 77% at 90 minutes, with no significant increase in bleeding (Figure 13.4). Myocardial perfusion, as assessed by ST-segment resolution, was also significantly improved.[33]

Although the rPA phase of the TIMI-14 trial as well as the Strategies for Patency Enhancement in the Emergency Department (SPEED) trial demonstrated that the combination of half-dose rPA (5 + 5 U) and abciximab demonstrated TIMI-3 flow in 63% of patients,[34] the recently completed GUSTO V trial demonstrated equivalent 30-day mortality outcomes between full dose rPA (5.9%) and half-dose rPA plus abciximab (5.6%). Reinfarction and urgent revascularization did occur less often with combination therapy.[40] The ASSENT-3 trial,[41] using a similar study design, demonstrated similar mortality outcomes in patients receiving full-dose TNK-tPA and reduced-dose unfractionated heparin (6%) and half-dose TNK-tPA plus abciximab (6.6%), with a trend toward lower mortality when enoxaparin was combined with TNK-tPA (5.4%) (Figure 13.5). However, patients in both trials over the age of 75 receiving the combination of a lytic agent and abciximab experienced a significant increase in intracranial bleeding.

The available data suggest that enhanced rates and extent of thrombolysis is achievable with combined pharmacotherapy; however, the safety and overall benefit can only be established through further investigation.

217

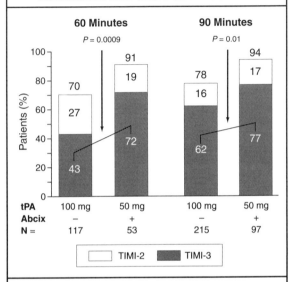

**FIGURE 13.4 — RESULTS FROM TIMI-14:
INFARCT ARTERY PATENCY FOLLOWING
ABCIXIMAB AND REDUCED-DOSE tPA**

Abbreviations: Abcix, abciximab; tPA, tissue plasminogen activator.

Results from the Thrombolysis in Myocardial Infarction 14 (TIMI-14) trial.

Antman et al. *Circulation*. 1999;99:2720-2732.

Heparin Preparations

Heparin is a naturally occurring inhibitor of thrombin, requiring formation of a ternary complex with antithrombin for an inhibitory effect. Several trials performed in the pre-reperfusion era demonstrated a 17% mortality reduction and a 22% reduction in risk of reinfarction with unfractionated heparin.[35]

These "historical" data, as well as the reduction in the incidence of venous thromboemboli, provided support for the use of IV UFH or subcutaneous low molecular weight heparin (LMWH) in patients with MI.[4,36]

218

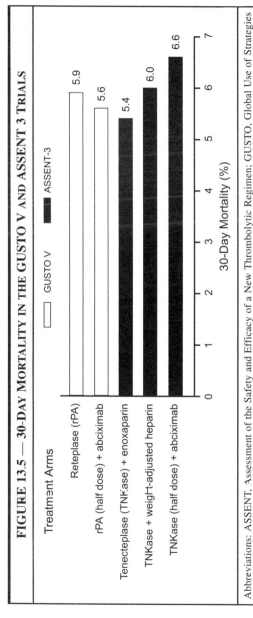

FIGURE 13.5 — 30-DAY MORTALITY IN THE GUSTO V AND ASSENT 3 TRIALS

□ GUSTO V   ■ ASSENT-3

Treatment Arms

Reteplase (rPA) — 5.9

rPA (half dose) + abciximab — 5.6

Tenecteplase (TNKase) + enoxaparin — 5.4

TNKase + weight-adjusted heparin — 6.0

TNKase (half dose) + abciximab — 6.6

30-Day Mortality (%)

Abbreviations: ASSENT, Assessment of the Safety and Efficacy of a New Thrombolytic Regimen; GUSTO, Global Use of Strategies to Open Occluded Arteries.

ASSENT-3 Investigators. Lancet. 2001;358:605-613; Topol EJ, the GUSTO V Investigators. Lancet. 2001;357:1905-1914.

13

Patients with an anterior infarction with anterior akinesis or dyskinesis, significant left ventricular dysfunction, left ventricular aneurysm, congestive heart failure, thrombus in the left ventricle documented by echocardiography, a history of a previous embolic event, and atrial fibrillation are at a high risk for systemic embolization[1] (Table 13.5). Although randomized trial data are sparse, there is evidence that the risk of systemic emboli can be reduced by early initiation of heparin therapy.[1] Therefore, independent of the fibrinolytic agent choice, heparin is recommended for patients at high risk for systemic embolism. Unless a contraindication exists, oral anticoagulant therapy with warfarin (target international normalized ratio [INR] 2.5) is continued for several months.

TABLE 13.5 — FACTORS THAT INCREASE THE RISK OF SYSTEMIC EMBOLIZATION FOLLOWING MYOCARDIAL INFARCTION

- Anterior infarction with anterior akinesis or dyskinesis
- Significant left ventricular dysfunction
- Acute left ventricular aneurysm
- Congestive heart failure
- Thrombus in the left ventricle documented by echocardiography
- History of a previous embolic event
- Atrial fibrillation

Patients receiving fibrin-selective agents, tPA, rPA, or TNK-tPA should receive weight-adjusted IV UFH (target activated partial thromboplastin time [aPTT] 50-70 sec) for 48 hours.[4] The dosing strategy is as follows: a 60-U/kg bolus at initiation of fibrinolytic therapy, followed by an initial maintenance dose of 12 U/kg/hr (maximum bolus of 4,000 U and a 1000 U/hr infusion in patients weighing >70 kg. If non–fibrin-selective fibrinolytics are used, such as SK or anistreplase, patients at low risk for thromboemboli can receive subcutaneous heparin, 7,500 to 10,000 U every 12 hours, until ambulatory.

Low Molecular Weight Heparin and Direct-Acting Antithrombins

Low molecular weight heparins provide several potential advantages over conventional UFH, owing to their improved bioavailability, enhanced antithrombotic effects mediated by "upstream" inhibition of the coagulation cascade and ease of use. Several trials are evaluating the role of LMWH as adjunctive antithrombotic therapy for patients receiving fibrinolytics.[4] As described, ASSENT-3 provided encouraging results for the combination of enoxaparin and TNK-tPA.[41] The National Investigators Collaboration on Enoxaparin (NICE) trials have demonstrated the safety and efficacy of enoxaparin in the catheterization laboratory during PCI, both with and without GPIIb/IIIa receptor antagonists.

Warfarin

A meta-analysis of trials performed in the pre-reperfusion era demonstrated that long-term oral anticoagulation was associated with a modest survival benefit of 20% in men, which was restricted to those with prolonged angina or previous MI.[1] The Warfarin Reinfarction Study (WARIS)[37] included patients with MI (mean 27 days from event) and randomized then to treatment with warfarin (target INR of 2.8 to 4.8), or placebo. There were statistically significant reductions in all-cause mortality (24%), reinfarction (34%), and stroke (55%) in favor of anticoagulant therapy.

The Coumadin Aspirin Reinfarction Study (CARS),[38] tested the efficacy of low-intensity anticoagulation with warfarin (1 mg/d to 3 mg/d) plus aspirin (80 mg/day) compared with aspirin alone (160 mg/day). Event rates were low and nearly identical in all three study arms of the trial. These results are consistent with a large body of literature that suggests that warfarin is most effective when given in doses capable of increasing the INR to 2 to 3.5 (moderate to high intensity anticoagulation).[1]

Oral anticoagulation with warfarin, titrated to a target INR of 2.5 represents a treatment option for several months following AMI in patients at high risk for venous or systemic thromboembolism (Table 13.5). Treatment is often initiated in the hospital, while the patient is still receiving IV or subcutaneous heparin. The availability of LMWH preparations that can be self-administered once or twice per day, provide a potential option for earlier hospital discharge with transition to warfarin therapy in the outpatient setting.

Summary

Acute thrombotic occlusion of an epicardial coronary artery, the most common cause of ST-segment elevation MI, is the end result of platelet activation and aggregation, followed by activation of the extrinsic and intrinsic pathways of coagulation. The clinician's antithrombotic armamentarium includes:

- Fibrinolytics used alone or as part of a facilitated strategy
- Mechanical techniques, such as immediate angioplasty and/or stenting, to restore perfusion and maintain patency
- Antiplatelet agents that inhibit platelet activation as well as aggregation through blockade of the GPIIb/IIIa receptor
- Antithrombotic compounds that prevent propagation of thrombus, particularly after successful reperfusion therapy.

Current research efforts are directed toward defining the safest and most efficacious pharmacological and mechanical treatments that achieve rapid and sustained patency of the infarct vessel, and limit subsequent atherothrombotic events.

REFERENCES

1. Cairns JA, Theroux P, Lewis HD Jr, Ezekowitz M, Meade TW. Antithrombotic agents in coronary artery disease. *Chest*. 2001; 119(suppl):228S-252S.

2. DeWood MA, Spores J, Notske R, et al. Prevalence of total coronary occlusion during the early hours of transmural myocardial infarction. *N Engl J Med*. 1980;303:897-902.

3. ISIS-2 (Second International Study of Infarct Survival) Collaborative Group. Randomised trial of intravenous streptokinase, oral aspirin, both, or neither among 17,187 cases of suspected acute myocardial infarction: ISIS-2. *Lancet*. 1988;2:349-360.

4. Ryan TJ, Antman EM, Brooks NH, et al. 1999 Update: ACC/AHA Guidelines for the management of patients with acute myocardial infarction. A report of the American College of Cardiology/American Heart Association Task Force on Practice Guidelines (Committee on Management of Acute Myocardial Infarction). *J Am Coll Cardiol*. 1999;34:890-911.

5. CAPRIE Steering Committee. A randomised, blinded, trial of clopidogrel versus aspirin in patients at risk of ischaemic events (CAPRIE). *Lancet*. 1996;348:1329-1339.

6. Sherry S. *Fibrinolysis, Thrombosis, and Hemostasis: Concepts, Perspectives, and Clinical Applications*. Philadelphia, Pa: Lea and Febiger; 1992:119-160.

7. Fibrinolytic Therapy Trialists' (FTT) Collaborative Group. Indications for fibrinolytic therapy in suspected acute myocardial infarction: collaborative overview of early mortality and major morbidity results from all randomised trials of more than 1000 patients [published correction appears in *Lancet*. 1994;343:742]. *Lancet*. 1994;343:311-322.

8. Late Assessment of Thrombolytic Efficacy (LATE) study with alteplase 6-24 hours after onset of acute myocardial infarction. *Lancet*. 1993;342:759-766.

9. EMERAS (Estudio Multicentrico Estreptoquinasa Republicas de America del Sur) Collaborative Group. Randomised trial of late thrombolysis in patients with suspected acute myocardial infarction. *Lancet*. 1993;342:767-772.

13

10. Gruppo Italiano per lo Studio della Sopravvivenza nell'Infarto Miocardico. GISSI-2: a factorial randomised trial of alteplase versus streptokinase and heparin versus no heparin among 12,490 patients with acute myocardial infarction. *Lancet*. 1990;336:65-71.

11. ISIS-3 (Third International Study of Infarct Survival) Collaborative Group. A randomised comparison of streptokinase vs tissue plasminogen activator vs anistreplase and of aspirin plus heparin vs aspirin alone among 41,299 cases of suspected acute myocardial infarction: ISIS-3. *Lancet*. 1992;339:753-770.

12. The GUSTO Investigators. An international randomized trial comparing four thrombolytic strategies for acute myocardial infarction. *N Engl J Med*. 1993;329:673-682.

13. The GUSTO Angiographic Investigators. The effects of tissue plasminogen activator, streptokinase, or both on coronary-artery patency, ventricular function, and survival after acute myocardial infarction. *N Engl J Med*. 1993;329:1615-1622.

14. Simes RJ, Topol EJ, Holmes DR Jr, et al, for the GUSTO-1 Investigators. Link between the angiographic substudy and mortality outcomes in a large randomized trial of myocardial reperfusion. Importance of early and complete infarct artery reperfusion. *Circulation*. 1995;91:1923-1928.

15. The Global Use of Strategies to Open Occluded Coronary Arteries (GUSTO III) Investigators. A comparison of reteplase with alteplase for acute myocardial infarction. *N Engl J Med*. 1997;337:1118-1123.

16. Cannon CP, Gibson CM, McCabe CH, et al. TNK-tissue plasminogen activator compared with front-loaded alteplase in acute myocardial infarction: results of the TIMI 10B trial. Thrombolysis in Myocardial Infarction (TIMI) 10B Investigators. *Circulation*. 1998; 98:2805-2814.

17. White HD, Van de Werf FJ. Thrombolysis for acute myocardial infarction. *Circulation*. 1998:97:1632-1646.

18. Gore JM, Granger CB, Simoons ML, et al. Stroke after thrombolysis. Mortality and functional outcomes in the GUSTO-I Trial. *Circulation*. 1995;92:2811-2818.

19. Cairns JA, Kennedy JW, Fuster V. Coronary thrombolysis. *Chest*. 1998:114(suppl):634S-657S.

20. Ross AM, Coyne KS, Reiner JS, et al. Randomized trial comparing angioplasty with a strategy of short acting thrombolysis and immediate planned rescue angioplasty in acute myocardial infarction: the PACT trial. *J Am Coll Cardiol*. 1999;34:1954-1962

21. Califf RM, O'Neil W, Stack RS, et al. Failure of simple clinical measurements to predict perfusion status after intravenous thrombolysis. *Ann Intern Med*. 1988;108:658-662.

22. Barron HV, Bowlby LJ, Breen T, et al. Use of reperfusion therapy for acute myocardial infarction in the United States: data from the National Registry of Myocardial Infarction 2. *Circulation*. 1998;97: 1150-1156.

23. Weaver WD, Simes RJ, Betriu A, et al. Comparison of primary coronary angioplasty and intravenous thrombolytic therapy for acute myocardial infarction: a quantitative review [published correction appears in *JAMA*. 1998;279:1876]. *JAMA*. 1997;278:2093-2098.

24. Michels KB, Yusuf S. Does PTCA in acute myocardial infarction affect mortality and reinfarction rates? A quantitative overview (meta-analysis) of the randomized clinical trials. *Circulation*. 1995;91:476-485.

25. The GUSTO IIb Angioplasty Substudy Investigators. A clinical trial comparing primary coronary angioplasty with tissue plasminogen activator for acute myocardial infarction [published correction appears in *N Engl J Med*. 1997;337:287]. *N Engl J Med*. 1997;336:1621-1628.

26. Tiefenbrunn AJ, Chandra NC, French WJ, Gore JM, Rogers WJ. Clinical experience with primary percutaneous transluminal coronary angioplasty compared with alteplase (recombinant tissue-type plasminogen activator) in patients with acute myocardial infarction: a report from the Second National Registry of Myocardial Infarction (NRMI-2). *J Am Coll Cardiol*. 1998;31:1240-1245.

27. Hochman JS, Sleeper LA, Webb JG, et al. Early revascularization in acute myocardial infarction complicated by cardiogenic shock. SHOCK Investigators. Should We Emergently Revascularize Occluded Coronaries for Cardiogenic Shock. *N Engl J Med*. 1999;341:625-634.

28. Moliterno DJ, Topol EJ. Conjunctive use of platelet glycoprotein IIb/IIIa antagonists and thrombolytic therapy for acute myocardial infarction. *Thromb Haemost*. 1997;78:214-219.

29. Cannon CP. Overcoming thrombolytic resistance. *J Am Coll Cardiol*. 1999;34:1395-1402.

30. Ito H, Okamura A, Isakura K, et al. Myocardial perfusion patterns related to immediate thrombolysis in myocardial infarction perfusion grades after coronary angioplasty in patients with acute anterior wall myocardial infarction. *Circulation*. 1996;93:1993-1999.

31. Brener S. Presentation of INTRO-AMI Data. AHA Scientific Sessions, November 1999.

32. Antman EM, Giugliano RP, Gibson CM, et al for the TIMI 14 Investigators. Abciximab facilitates the rate and extent of thrombolysis: results of TIMI-14 trial. *Circulation*. 1999;99:2720-2732.

33. de Lemos JA, Antman EM, Gibson CM, et al. Abciximab improves both epicardial flow and myocardial reperfusion in ST elevation myocardial infarction: a TIMI 14 analysis. *Circulation*. In press.

34. Ohman EM, Lincoff AM, Boode C, et al. Enhanced early reperfusion at 60 minutes with low-dose reteplase combined with full-dose abciximab in acute myocardial infarction: preliminary results from the GUSTO-4 pilot (SPEED) dose-ranging trial. *Circulation*. 1998;98(suppl 1):I-504. Abstract.

35. MacMahon S, Collins R, Knight C, Yusuf S, Peto R. Reduction in major morbidity and mortality by heparin in acute myocardial infarction. *Circulation*. 1988;78:(supp 2):II-98. Abstract.

13

36. Rao AK, Pratt C, Berke A, et al. Thrombolysis in Myocardial Infarction (TIMI) Trial—phase I: hemorrhagic manifestations and changes in plasma fibrinogen and the fibrinolytic system in patients treated with recombinant tissue plasminogen activator and streptokinase. *J Am Coll Cardiol*. 1988;11:1-11.

37. Smith P, Arnesen H, Holme I. The effect of warfarin on mortality and reinfarction after myocardial infarction. *N Engl J Med*. 1990;323:147-152.

38. Coumadin Aspirin Reinfarction Study (CARS) Investigators. Randomized, double-blind trial of fixed low dose warfarin with aspirin after myocardial infarction. *Lancet*. 1997;350:389-396.

39. The Clopiogrel in Unstable Angina to Prevent Recurrent Events (CURE) Trial Investigators: Effects of clopidogrel in addition to aspirin in patients with acute coronary syndromes without ST-segment elevation. *N Engl J Med*. 2001;345:494-502.

40. Topol EJ, The GUSTO V Investigators. Reperfusion therapy for acute myocardial infarction with fibrinolytic therapy or combination reduced fibrinolytic therapy and platelet glycoprotein IIb/IIIa inhibition: the GUSTO V randomised trial. *Lancet*. 2001;357:1905-1914.

41. The Assessment of the Safety and Efficacy of a New Thrombolytic Regimen (ASSENT)-3 Investigators. Efficacy and safety of tenecteplase in combination with enoxaparin, abciximab, or unfractionated heparin: the ASSENT-3 randomised trial in acute myocardial infarction. *Lancet*. 2001;358:605-613.

14

Noncardiac Arterial Disease: Peripheral Arterial Vascular Disease and Stroke

Vascular disease of the peripheral arterial circulation, most often caused by atherosclerosis and less commonly by vasculitis (or other nonatherosclerotic arteriopathies), is a chronic process that is responsible for progressive and, at times, incapacitating symptoms, disability, and limb loss. The arterial beds most frequently involved, in order of occurrence, are:

- Femoro-popliteal-tibial
- Aortoiliac
- Carotid and vertebral
- Splanchnic and renal
- Brachiocephalic.

The causes of acute occlusion include:

- Cardioembolism
- Artery-to-artery embolism
- In situ thrombosis
- Trauma.
- Vasospasm.

The frequent coexistence of peripheral vascular and coronary artery disease (multi-bed vascular disease) has been recognized for decades and is clinically important for several reasons. First, it provides a unifying basis for atherosclerosis and its prevention. Second, it offers a biologically plausible explanation for the high cardiovascular mortality (two- to threefold increase) in patients with peripheral vascular disease. Last, the pharmacologic approach to management takes on a more global theme with the objective of preventing atherosclerosis progression and attenuating thrombotic processes, which underlie acute myocardial infarction (MI), stroke, and peripheral arterial occlusion (Figure 14.1).

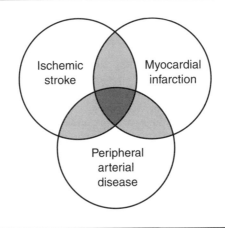

FIGURE 14.1 — THROMBOTIC PROCESSES ASSOCIATED WITH ATHEROSCLEROSIS PROGRESSION

Ischemic stroke

Myocardial infarction

Peripheral arterial disease

Atherosclerosis is a generalized or "multi-bed" process that typically involves the peripheral, coronary, and cerebral vasculature.

Vascular Disease

The available data, derived from individual clinical trials and from a frequently cited meta-analysis conducted by the Antiplatelet Trialists' Collaboration, provide strong support for therapies targeting platelet inhibition among patients with vascular disease. In high-risk patients, aspirin therapy (80 mg to 325 mg qd) reduced nonfatal MI by one third, nonfatal stroke by one third, and death from all vascular causes by one sixth.[1] The benefit applies to a broad range of individuals, including men and women of all ages and those with hypertension or diabetes mellitus.

Cerebrovascular Disease

Ischemic stroke is a major cause of morbidity and mortality worldwide and, in a large proportion of patients, is caused by atherosclerosis involving the carotid (extracranial) and cerebral (intracranial) vasculature. The benefit of platelet antagonists in patients with prior stroke or transient ischemic attack has been documented by several large-scale clinical trials (Table 14.1) and in an overview of all previously conducted trials.[1-10] Ticlopidine (or clopidogrel) may offer additional benefit (compared with aspirin) in patients with a recent stroke or fixed neurologic defect, reducing the occurrence of fatal or nonfatal stroke by 15% to 20%;[5] however, side effects (including neutropenia) are a concern with long-term administration of ticlopidine. Combined aspirin and dipyridamole preparations (Aggrenox) may offer benefit.

The primary prevention of stroke with pharmacologic therapy (predominantly platelet antagonists) while efficacious has limitations. Patients with advanced carotid disease (stenosis >70%) remain at risk for neurologic events and should be considered for carotid endarterectomy; however, antiplatelet therapy should be continued postoperatively. Anticoagulant therapy with warfarin is preferable following cardioembolic stroke, particularly in the setting of atrial fibrillation.

Peripheral Occlusive Disease

Patients with peripheral vascular (occlusive) disease have specific needs that reflect the disseminated nature of atherosclerosis. Intermittent claudication is a manifestation of ischemic muscle that reflects a fixed obstruction to blood flow and periods of heightened intravascular thrombotic activity.

Because of its dynamic pathobiology and clinical expression, the treatment of patients with peripheral vascular disease has included lifestyle changes (risk-factor modification), vasoactive compounds, muscle-metabolism enhancing drugs, and antithrombotic therapy (aspirin, clopidogrel, or their combination).[12-16]

Critical limb ischemia, as a distinct clinical entity, represents the progression of ischemia to the point of severely compromised nutritive blood flow that threatens tissue viability. The manifestations range from claudication at rest to trophic skin changes and ulceration to overt gangrene and limb loss. Although revascularization represents the treatment of choice, this is not always feasible, raising the ques-

TABLE 14.1 — RANDOMIZED TRIALS IN PATIENTS WITH EITHER ISCHEMIC STROKE OR TRANSIENT ISCHEMIC ATTACKS RECEIVING PLATELET ANTAGONIST THERAPY

Trial	Patients	Treatment	Comparison(s)	Clinical Outcome(s)	Findings
CAPRIE (1997)	19,185	• Clopidogrel 75 mg qd • Peripheral arterial disease, recent stroke, recent MI	• ASA 325 mg qd	• Ischemic stroke, MI, or vascular death • Stroke • GIH	• PAD patients: RRR 23.8% ($P = 0.0028$) • RRR 7.3% ($P = 0.26$) • 0.52% vs. 0.93% ($P < 0.05$)
CAST (1997)	21,106	• ASA 160 mg qd within 48 h	• Placebo	• Mortality • Death or nonfatal stroke	• 3.3% vs 3.9%; OR 14%; $P = 0.004$ • 5.3% vs 5.9%; OR 12%; $P = 0.03$
IST (1997)	19,435	• ASA 300 mg qd within 48 h	• SQ heparin • SQ heparin + ASA • Neither	• Mortality at 14 days • Recurrent stroke • Death or dependence at 6 mo	• 9.0% vs 9.4%; not significant • 2.8% vs 3.9%; $P < 0.001$ • Not significant
ESPS-2 (1996)	6,062	• ASA 25 mg bid, dipyridamole 200 mg bid, ASA + dipyridamole* • TIA or completed ischemic stroke within 2 mo	• Placebo	• Mortality • Recurrent stroke	• No difference • ASA RRR 18% ($P = 0.013$) • Dipyridamole RRR 16% ($P = 0.039$) • ASA + dipyridamole RRR 37% ($P < 0.001$)
MAST-I (1995)	622	• ASA 300 mg within 6 h	• Untreated • Streptokinase • ASA + streptokinase	• Mortality	• OR 2.7 (1.7–4.3) streptokinase • OR 0.9 (0.6–1.3) ASA + streptokinase

SALT (1991)	1,360	• ASA 75 mg qd 1 to 4 mo after cerebrovascular event	—	• Mortality • Stroke • Bleeding event	• 18% RRR • 18% RRR • 7.2% vs 3.2%; $P = 0.001$
UK-TIA 1991	1,072	• ASA 300 mg qd, ASA 600 mg bid	• Placebo	• Mortality • GI bleeding	• 15% RRR (−3%–29%) • 3.3% with 300 mg; 6.4% with 1200 mg
CATS (1989)	1,072	• Ticlopidine 250 mg bid • Recent thromboembolic stroke	• Placebo	• Stroke, MI, vascular death • As above, but intent-to-treat • Stroke, stroke-related death • Severe side effects	• RRR 30.2% • RRR 23.3%: $P = 0.02$ • RRR 24.1% • 8.2% vs 2.8%
TASS (1989)	3,069	• Ticlopidine 250 mg bid • TIA, anaurosis fugax, RIND, minor stroke within 3 mo	• ASA 650 mg bid	• Nonfatal stroke, death • Fatal stroke, nonfatal stroke • Severe neutropenia	• 17% vs 19%; RRR 12%; −2%–26% • 10% vs 13%; RRR 21%; 4%–38% • 13/1529 vs 0/1540

Abbreviations: ASA, aspirin; CAPRIE, Clopidogrel vs Aspirin in Patients at Risk for Ischemic Events; CAST, Chinese Acute Stroke Trial; CATS, Canadian-American Ticlodipine Study; ESPS, European Stroke Prevention Study; GI, gastrointestinal; GIH, gastrointestinal hemorrhage; IST, International Stroke Trial; MAST, Multicenter Acute Stroke Trial; MI, myocardial infarction; OR, odds ratio; PAD, peripheral arterial disease; RIND, reversible ischemic neurologic deficit; RRR, relative risk reduction; SALT, Swedish Aspirin Low-Dose Trial; SQ, subcutaneous; TASS, Ticlopidine Aspirin Stroke Study; TIA, transient ischemic attack; UK-TIA, United Kingdom Transient Ischemic Attack.

* Extended-release preparation.

14

tion of pharmacologic alternatives. A majority of clinical trials performed to date have focused on vasodilating compounds like cilostazol, many of which also possess antithrombotic properties.[17-21]

Acute Arterial Insufficiency

The predominant causes of acute arterial insufficiency are trauma, in situ thrombosis, and peripheral embolism. Nontraumatic occlusion can be further classified as thrombotic or embolic. The former is typically associated with advanced atherosclerosis and most often involves the lower extremities. In approximately 85% of cases, arterial embolism originates within the heart (atrial fibrillation, valvular heart disease, left ventricular mural thrombus). Noncardiac sources include abdominal aortic or femoral aneurysms, ulcerated atherosclerotic plaques, and paradoxic emboli from lower-extremity venous thrombi that cross into the arterial circulation through atrial septal defects, patent foramen ovale, or ventricular septal defects. The most common sites of involvement in descending order of frequency include the iliofemoral, popliteal, and tibial vessels. Diagnostic hallmarks of arterial occlusion are sudden pain with pallor, loss of pulse, and paresthesias. Prolonged ischemia can lead to sensory and motor loss and ultimately tissue necrosis (gangrene).

Acute peripheral emboli are frequently managed with balloon extraction and systemic anticoagulation. The role of anticoagulant therapy (most often with unfractionated heparin [UFH]) is to prevent recurrent cardio- and artery-to-artery embolization. It may also reduce in situ thrombosis in areas of endothelial disruption created by the original thrombus and/or balloon extraction-related trauma. Distal (popliteal artery and below) emboli and acute thrombotic occlusion can be managed with either surgery or selective intra-arterial fibrinolytic therapy. Although a consensus has not been reached, fibrinolytic therapy may be most useful in surgically inaccessible small arteries of the forearm, hand, leg, and foot and in patients who are not considered candidates for surgical intervention.[22] The adjunctive role of platelet glycoprotein (GP) IIb/IIIa antagonists is under investigation, but should be considered with recurring thrombosis despite adequate anticoagulation.

A reduction in cardiovascular events, including MI and vascular death, is a primary goal of antithrombotic therapy in patients with peripheral vascular disease. The Antiplatelet Trialists Collaboration overview[1] documented the benefit of antiplatelet therapy in this subset defined as having either intermittent claudication, peripheral bypass grafts, or peripheral angioplasty. The question that most clinicians ask is "What is the preferred antagonist?" Aspirin or clopidogrel is accepted therapy with the latter representing a preferable treatment strategy in patients with peripheral vascular disease and known coronary artery disease (dual vascular bed disease)[2] (Figure 14.2). The potential for added benefit with combined strategies of aspirin and clopidogrel has been confirmed with coronary artery disease.

Peripheral Vascular Reconstructive Surgery

Although the available literature suggests that saphenous veins have patency rates that are superior to polytetrafluoroethylene bypass grafts, both are subject to early thrombotic occlusion that stems from in situ thrombogenicity, technical challenges and, in many patients, poor distal runoff. The importance of flow is highlighted by the comparatively low rates of occlusion involving arteries greater than 6 mm in diameter (aortoiliac, femoral) compared with smaller vessels and flow rates less than 200 mL/minute. Although intermediate and late occlusions may also be thrombotic in origin, neointimal hyperplasia and progressive atherosclerosis dominate the pathobiology.[23,24]

Because the platelets represent the predominant constituent of arterial thrombi, antiplatelet therapy with aspirin or clopidogrel is considered the standard of care for patients undergoing reconstructive procedures (or angioplasty). Systemic anticoagulation with UFH may be protective at the time of intraoperative vessel cross-clamping. The combination of warfarin and aspirin (or an alternative platelet antagonist) should be reserved for high-risk patients (poor vein quality, marginal arterial runoff, and previously failed bypass).[25]

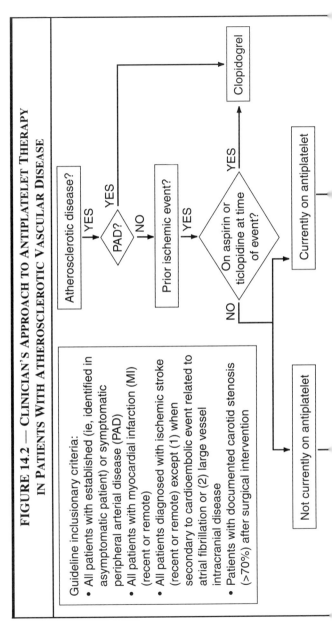

FIGURE 14.2 — CLINICIAN'S APPROACH TO ANTIPLATELET THERAPY IN PATIENTS WITH ATHEROSCLEROTIC VASCULAR DISEASE

Atherosclerotic disease?

YES

PAD? — YES → Clopidogrel

NO

Prior ischemic event?

YES

On aspirin or ticlopidine at time of event?

YES → Clopidogrel

NO

Currently on antiplatelet

Not currently on antiplatelet

Guideline inclusionary criteria:

- All patients with established (ie, identified in asymptomatic patient) or symptomatic peripheral arterial disease (PAD)
- All patients with myocardial infarction (MI) (recent or remote)
- All patients diagnosed with ischemic stroke (recent or remote) except (1) when secondary to cardioembolic event related to atrial fibrillation or (2) large vessel intracranial disease
- Patients with documented carotid stenosis (>70%) after surgical intervention

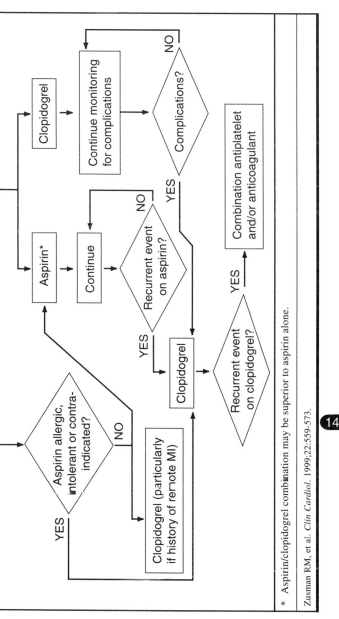

Aspirin allergic, intolerant or contra-indicated?

YES → Clopidogrel (particularly if history of remote MI)

NO → Aspirin*

Aspirin* → Continue

Continue → Recurrent event on aspirin?

NO (continue)

YES → Clopidogrel

Clopidogrel → Recurrent event on clopidogrel?

YES → Combination antiplatelet and/or anticoagulant

Clopidogrel → Continue monitoring for complications

Continue monitoring for complications → Complications?

NO

YES → Combination antiplatelet and/or anticoagulant

* Aspirin/clopidogrel combination may be superior to aspirin alone.

Zusman RM, et al. *Clin Cardiol.* 1999;22:559-573.

14

Summary

Atherosclerosis is a systemic inflammatory disease that commonly involves a variety of vascular beds. Patients with peripheral vascular disease, in addition to experiencing ischemic symptoms (claudication) are at risk for limb loss, stroke, MI, and cardiovascular death (Table 14.2).[26] Risk-factor modification takes on a global purpose in these patients; antithrombotic therapy, by preventing acute thrombotic events, plays a vital protective role. Aspirin (81 mg/d to 325 mg/d) or clopidogrel (75 mg/d) should be administered to those with a prior MI or documented multi-bed vascular disease.

REFERENCES

1. Antiplatelet Trialists Collaboration. Secondary prevention of vascular disease by prolonged antiplatelet treatment. *Br Med J.* 1988;296:320-331.

2. CAPRIE Steering Committee. A randomised, blinded trial of clopidogrel versus aspirin in patients at risk of ischaemic events (CAPRIE). *Lancet.* 1996;348:1329-1339.

3. CAST (Chinese Acute Stroke Trial) Collaborative Group. CAST: randomised placebo-controlled trial of early aspirin use in 20,000 patients with acute ischaemic stroke. *Lancet.* 1997;349:1641-1649.

4. International Stroke Trial Collaborative Group. The International Stroke Trial (IST): a randomised trial of aspirin, subcutaneous heparin, both, or neither among 19,435 patients with acute ischaemic stroke. *Lancet.* 1997;349:1569-1581.

5. Hass WK, Easton JD, Adams HP, et al. A randomized trial comparing ticlopidine hydrochloride with aspirin for the prevention of stroke in high-risk patients. Ticlopidine Aspirin Stroke Study Group. *N Engl J Med.* 1989;321:501-507.

6. Gent M, Blakely JA, Easton JD, et al. The Canadian American Ticlopidine Study (CATS) in thromboembolic stroke. *Lancet.* 1989;1:1215-1220.

7. Diener HC, Cunha L, Forbes C, Sivenius J, Smets P, Lowenthal A. European Stroke Prevention Study. 2. Dipyridamole and acetylsalicylic acid in the secondary prevention of stroke. *J Neurol Sci.* 1996;143:1-13.

8. Multicentre Acute Stroke Trial – Italy (MAST-I) Group. Randomised controlled trial of streptokinase, aspirin, and combination of both in treatment of acute ischaemic stroke. *Lancet*. 1995;346:1509-1514.

9. The SALT Collaborative Group. Swedish Aspirin Low-Dose Trial (SALT) of 75 mg aspirin as secondary prophylaxis after cerebrovascular ischaemic events. *Lancet*. 1991;338:1345-1349.

10. Farrell B, Godwin J, Richards S, Warlow C. The United Kingdom transient ischaemic attack (UK-TIA) aspirin trial: final results. *J Neurol Neurosurg Psychiatry*. 1991;54:1044-1054.

11. Lindgarde F, Jelnes R, Bjorkman H, et al, for the Scandinavian Study Group. Conservative drug treatment in patients with moderately severe chronic occlusive peripheral arterial disease. *Circulation*. 1989; 80:1549-1556.

12. Balsano F, Coccheri S, Libretti A, et al. Ticlopidine in the treatment of intermittent claudication: a 21-month double-blind trial. *J Lab Clin Med*. 1989;114:84-91.

13. Ernst E, Kollar L, Matrai A. A double-blind trial of Dextran— haemodilution vs placebo in claudicants. *J Intern Med*. 1990;227:19-24.

14. Brevetti G, Perna S, Sabba C, Martone VD, Condorelli M. Propionyl-L-carnitine in intermittent claudication: double-blind, placebo-controlled, dose titration, multicenter study. *J Am Coll Cardiol*. 1995;26: 1411-1416.

15. Belch JJ, Bell PR, Creissen D, et al. Randomized, double-blind, placebo-controlled study evaluating the efficacy and safety of AS-013, a prostaglandin E_1 prodrug, in patients with intermittent claudication. *Circulation*. 1997;95:2298-2302.

16. Liervre M, Azoulay S, Lion L, Morand S, Girre JP, Boissel JP. A dose-effect study of beraprost sodium in intermittent claudication. *J Cardiovasc Pharmacol*. 1996;27:788-793.

17. Ciprostene Study Group. The effect of ciprostene in patients with peripheral vascular disease (PVD) characterized by ischemic ulcers. *J Clin Pharmacol*. 1991;31;81-87.

18. Diehm C, Balzer K, Bisler H, et al. Efficacy of a new prostaglandin E_1 regimen in outpatients with severe, intermittent claudication: results of a multicenter placebo-controlled double-blind trial. *J Vasc Surg*. 1997;256:537-544.

19. Norgren L, Alwmark A, Angqvist KA, et al. A stable prostacyclin analogue (iloprost) in the treatment of ischaemic ulcers of the lower limb. A Scandinavian-Polish placebo controlled, randomised multicenter study. *Eur J Vasc Surg*. 1990;4:463-467.

14

Clinical Scenario	Agent	Dosing Range/Comments
Carotid endarterectomy	Aspirin	81-325 mg/d
Prior transient ischemic attack	Aspirin	50-325 mg/d
	Aspirin/persantine	25/200 mg bid
	Clopidogrel	75 mg/d
Acute arterial occlusion/ischemia	Unfractionated heparin*	aPTT 2 × control
	Fibrinolytic therapy	tPA
Chronic lower extremity ischemia	Aspirin	81-325 mg/d
	Clopidogrel†	75 mg/d
Claudication	Aspirin	81-325 mg/d
	Clopidogrel	75 mg/d
	Cilostazol	50-100 mg bid

TABLE 14.2 — ANTITHROMBOTIC THERAPY IN PERIPHERAL VASCULAR DISEASE

Intraoperative anticoagulation during vascular surgery	Unfractionated heparin	aPTT 2-3 × control
Infrainguinal vein bypass	Aspirin	81-325 mg/d
	Clopidogrel	75 mg/d (if aspirin not used)
Infrainguinal prosthetic bypass	Aspirin	81-325 mg/d
Infrainguinal bypass (high thrombotic risk)	Aspirin plus warfarin	81-325 mg/d; INR 2.5 (range 2.0-3.0)
Aortoiliac or renal PCI	Aspirin	325 mg/d
	Clopidogrel	75 mg/d (stenting)

Abbreviations: aPTT, activated partial thromboplastin time; INR, international normalized ratio; PCI, percutaneous coronary intervention; tPA, tissue plasminogen activator.

* Followed by warfarin to INR 2.5 (range 2.0-3.0).
† Clopidogrel may be superior to aspirin for reducing vascular complications.

14

20. United Kingdom Severe Limb Ischemia Study Group. Treatment of limb threatening ischaemia with intravenous iloprost: a randomised double-blind placebo controlled study. *Eur J Vasc Surg.* 1991;5:511-516.

21. Guilmot JL, Diot E for the French Iloprost Study Group. Treatment of lower limb ischamia due to atherosclerosis in diabetic and non-diabetic patients with iloprost, a stable analogue of prostacyclin: results of a French Multicentre trial. *Drug Invest.* 1991;3:351-359.

22. STILE Investigators. Results of a prospective randomized trial evaluating surgery versus thrombolysis for ischemia of the lower extremity. *Ann Surg.* 1994;220:251-268.

23. Eickhoff JH, Buchardt Hansen HJ, Bromme A, et al. A randomized clinical trial of PTFE versus human umbilical vein for femoropopliteal bypass surgery. Preliminary results. *Br J Surg.* 1983;70:85-88.

24. McCollum C, Kenchington G, Alexander C, Franks PJ, Greenhalgh RM. PTFE or HUV for femoro-popliteal bypass: a multi-centre trial. *Eur J Vasc Surg.* 1991;5:435-443.

25. Sarac TP, Huber TS, Back MR, et al. Warfarin improves the outcome of infrainguinal vein bypass grafts at high risk for failure. *J Vasc Surg.* 1998;28:446-457.

26. The sixth (2000) ACCP guidelines for antithrombotic therapy for prevention and treatment of thrombosis. *Chest.* 2001;119(suppl):1S-370S.

27. Sakaguchi S. Prostaglandin E_1 intra-arterial infusion therapy in patients with ischemic ulcer of the extremities. *Int Angiol.* 1984:3:39-42.

15 Native and Prosthetic Valvular Heart Disease

Scope of the Problem

There are an estimated 250,000 heart valve replacement surgeries performed yearly on a worldwide basis. Mechanical prosthesis have an excellent track record of durability (25 years or more), but require lifelong anticoagulation. Improved hemodynamics and reduced thrombogenecity characterize bioprosthetic valves; however, there is the disadvantage of degeneration, particularly in younger individuals. The ideal replacement—a tissue engineered "copy" of a native valve—is decades away in development.

The most feared and devastating complication of native or prosthetic valvular heart disease for patients, clinicians, and surgeons alike is systemic embolism. Although the incidence of thromboembolic events has decreased in North America in parallel with the reduced occurrence of rheumatic heart disease, this has not been the case in other parts of the world. Moreover, despite the improvements in design and surgical technique, thromboembolism remains a serious complication of prosthetic heart valve replacement.

Mechanisms

Clinical, pathologic, and experimental evidence supports two predominant mechanisms for the initiation of thrombosis in patients with native or prosthetic valvular heart disease. The first involves disruption of the vascular endothelial surface and exposure of underlying prothrombotic substrate and/or the introduction of prothrombotic materials into the circulation. The second is mediated by "triggering" of thrombosis in areas of stasis. Early observations established that stasis alone required prolonged periods of time to induce thrombosis; however, the combination of stasis and localized tissue abnormalities and/or a high concentration of coagulation factors is profoundly

15

thrombogenic.[1-3] There is also evidence that prolonged periods of stasis impair tissue perfusion, with resulting endovascular damage and compromised fibrinolytic activity. Extension of thrombus into regions of relative stasis is common and represents an important mechanism for thrombus growth following prosthetic heart valve surgery.[4]

Natural History of Valvular Thrombi

The potential fate of thrombi formed within the cardiovascular system, including those associated with native and prosthetic valvular heart disease, includes:
- Partial or complete lysis
- Organization
- Partial organization with the potential for embolization.

Freshly formed fibrin strands are the most susceptible to lysis. Organization typically begins within 48 hours and is characterized by reduced concentrations of platelets, fibrin, and neutrophils, with a gradual replacement by monocytes, phagocytic cells, and fibroblasts during the first week and smooth muscle cells and connective tissue matrix during the second week. The last step in reducing thrombogenicity, and one of particular importance, is reendothelialization. As a rule, thrombi formed at sites of inflammation and injury organize more rapidly than stasis-related thrombi.[5,6]

Endothelial cells grow from the point of junction between a prosthetic valve and host tissue. Most believe that endothelium grows to confluence on the prosthetic valve surface, reducing the intermediate and long-term risk of thromboembolism.[7,8] It is clear, however, that despite the important thromboresistant properties of endothelial cells, prosthetic heart valves remain thrombogenic, certainly more so than native valves. This emphasizes the importance of blood flow geometry (high and low shear stress, stasis) as a major contributing factor in thrombogenesis and raises a question of chronic endothelial/neoendothelial cell injury or dysfunction as a lingering risk factor.

Prosthetic Heart Valve Thrombosis

The prerequisite conditions for prosthetic heart valve thrombosis can be defined conceptually in the context of Virchow's triad, with modifications for the introduction of a fourth component, an artificial surface. The traditional and widely cited components—abnormalities of the vascular/endothelial surface, stasis of blood flow, and abnormalities within the circulating blood—are all operational in the setting of prosthetic mechanical heart valve replacement.

The overall "thrombogenic surface" of prosthetic heart valves includes not only the artificial material itself but also the perivalvular excision tissue, sewing ring, and sutures as well. Each element is important, particularly in the early postoperative period when blood flow is reinitiated and the prothrombotic effects of surgery (platelet activation, circulating inflammatory mediators) are at their peak.

Blood flow across the aortic valve is typically rapid and characterized by regions of acceleration and high shear stress. Under these conditions, platelets are activated and erythrocyte membranes are damaged, leading to the release of adenosine diphosphate, further platelet activation, and ultimately, aggregation. The contribution of coagulation factors to overall thrombotic potential is a *secondary phenomenon* (Figure 15.1). In contrast, blood flow across the mitral valve is comparatively slow, particularly with coexistent mitral stenosis accompanied by left atrial enlargement or long-standing mitral insufficiency and left ventricular dilatation (Figure 15.2). In these settings, coagulation factor activation and interactions with the chamber walls and prosthetic material are the *primary phenomena* favoring thrombus formation, while platelets play a supportive role.

Tissue (bioprosthetic) valves, particularly those placed in the aortic position, often enjoy central unimpeded (laminar) blood flow without regions of either stagnation or acceleration. Although the cloth-covered stent and sewing ring are thrombogenic, the risk of thromboembolism is low, averaging 1% per patient year, and of concern only for the first 3 postoperative months before an organized neointima has developed. In the mitral position, the incidence of arterial thromboembolism is increased two- to threefold, based

15

FIGURE 15.1 — CHARACTERISTICS OF BLOOD FLOW ACROSS THE AORTIC VALVE

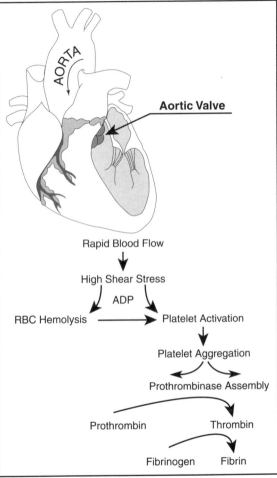

Blood flow across the aortic valve (native or prosthetic) is rapid and characterized by high shear stress, leading to platelet activation (direct and indirect via adenosine diphosphate [ADP] released from hemolyzed red blood cells [RBC]). Thus platelets play a central role in thrombogenicity, while coagulation factors serve in a supportive capacity for thrombus growth.

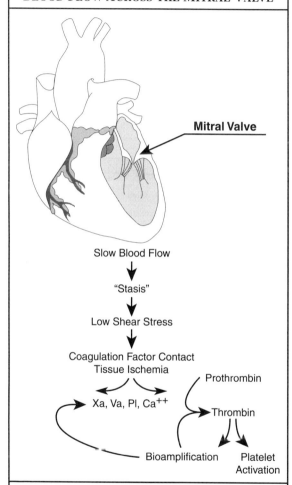

FIGURE 15.2 — CHARACTERISTICS OF BLOOD FLOW ACROSS THE MITRAL VALVE

Mitral Valve

Slow Blood Flow
↓
"Stasis"
↓
Low Shear Stress
↓
Coagulation Factor Contact
Tissue Ischemia

Xa, Va, Pl, Ca^{++}

Prothrombin

Thrombin

Bioamplification

Platelet Activation

Blood flow across the mitral valve, particularly with concomitant left atrial enlargement and reduced left ventricular performance, is slow or "static." Contact activation of clotting factors represents the primary mechanism of enhanced thrombogenicity, with thrombin-mediated platelet activation playing a supporting role.

15

predominantly on the high incidence of concomitant left atrial enlargement, atrial fibrillation, prior thromboembolism, and reduced left ventricular performance.[9,10]

Mechanical prosthetic heart valves, although more thrombogenic than tissue valves, are also more durable. Technical improvements in prosthesis design and the development of less thrombogenic materials have reduced the risk of thrombotic complications, which, at the present time, occur at an incidence of 3% to 5% per patient year.[11] Similar to tissue valves, mechanical heart valves in the mitral position are associated with a greater risk of thromboembolism than those in the aortic position.[12-14]

Assessing Thromboembolic Risk

■ **Native Valvular Heart Disease**

The risk of thromboembolism in patients with native valvular heart disease is influenced strongly by the site of involvement, chamber dimension, ventricular performance, and the presence of concomitant risk factors such as atrial fibrillation. Prior thromboembolism is considered a strong risk factor for recurrent events regardless of the valvular pathology.

■ **Clinical Experience**

The risk of thromboembolism in patients with prosthetic valvular heart disease is recognized. Despite methodologic limitations, the available information derived from relatively large studies and an ever-expanding clinical experience allows several conclusions to be drawn:

- Thromboprophylaxis for mechanical prostheses is achieved most effectively with oral anticoagulants.
- Antiplatelet therapy *alone* does not offer adequate protection for patients with mechanical prostheses.
- The thrombogenicity of mechanical heart valves, from greatest to least, is as follows: caged ball > tilting disk > bileaflet.
- High-risk patients (increased risk for thromboembolism) benefit from combination (anticoagulant and platelet antagonist) antithrombotic therapy.
- A "threshold" level of anticoagulation is required for benefit.

- High intensity anticoagulation (international normalized ratio [INR] >3.5) increases the risk for hemorrhagic complications.
- The risk of thromboembolism following bioprosthetic heart valve replacement is greatest during the first 3 postoperative months.[15-20]

Risk Stratification

The management of patients with native and prosthetic valvular heart disease must be approached comprehensively, taking into consideration not only the valve itself but the "company that it keeps" as well. Risk stratification, although focused predominantly on the "thrombotic side" of the equation, must be balanced to include the potential risk of hemorrhage with systemic anticoagulant therapy, particularly in patients with valvular heart disease in whom surgical procedures are being considered[21] (Tables 15.1 and 15.2).

Anticoagulant Therapy: Recommendations and Management Guidelines

The recommended approach to patients with native and prosthetic valvular heart disease is based on a composite of clinical trial results and clinical experience,[22] the latter is particularly true of native valvular disease for which few randomized clinical trials have been conducted (Tables 15.3, 15.4, and 15.5).

Early Postoperative Anticoagulant Therapy

15

Owing to the paucity of clinical trials, early postoperative anticoagulant therapy has been approached in a variety of ways. Low-dose systemic anticoagulation with either unfractionated heparin or low molecular weight heparin should be instituted once hemostasis has been secured and the risk for thrombosis outweighs the risk of hemorrhage. Unless the clinical conditions dictate otherwise, he-

TABLE 15.1 — THOMBOEMBOLIC RISK SCALE

Low-Risk*
- Atrial fibrillation
- Bioprosthetic heart valve (>3 months post-op)
- St. Jude mechanical heart valve (aortic position) (>6 months post-op)
- Dilated cardiomyopathy (ejection fraction <35%)

Intermediate-Risk
- Atrial fibrillation and prior thromboembolism (>3 months)
- St. Jude mechanical heart valve (aortic position) plus atrial fibrillation or ejection fraction <35%
- Dilated cardiomyopathy and prior thromboembolism (>3 months)
- Two low-risk factors
- Anterior myocardial infarction <3 months (no other risk factors)
- St. Jude mechanical heart valve ≤6 months post-op or in mitral position
- Bjork-Shiley (tilting disk) mechanical heart valve (aortic position)

High-Risk
- Atrial fibrillation and prior thromboembolism (<3 months)
- Dilated cardiomyopathy and prior thromboembolism (<3 months)
- Bjork-Shiley mechanical heart valve (mitral position) and any other risk factor
- St. Jude mechanical heart valve (aortic position) and ≥1 intermediate-risk factor
- Caged-ball mechanical heart valve (mitral position)

Very High-Risk
- Antiphospholipid antibody syndrome plus prior event or additional risk factors
- Cardioversion ≤2 weeks
- Arterial thromboembolic event ≤1 month
- Caged-ball mechanical heart valve (any position) plus additional risk factors
- Any combination of ≥2 risk factors

* Any of the low-risk factors plus *no* prior thromboembolism.

UMASS-Memorial Medical Center. 2001.

TABLE 15.2 — HEMORRHAGIC RISK SCALE

Low-Risk
- Dental procedures*
- Cataract surgery
- Angiography (diagnostic)
- Cystoscopy
- Breast biopsy
- Arthroscopic surgery

Intermediate-Risk
- Total hip replacement
- Total knee replacement
- Laparoscopic surgery
- Maxillofacial surgery
- Transurethral prostate removal
- Hysterectomy
- Colonoscopy with biopsy
- Prostate biopsy
- Skin graft

High-Risk
- Major abdominal surgery
- Major thoracic surgery
- Brain/central nervous system surgery
- Radical prostatectomy
- Skin graft
- Liver biopsy
- Kidney biopsy

* Exception: multiple extractions.

UMASS-Memorial Medical Center. 2001.

parin should be continued until adequate anticoagulation with warfarin has been achieved.

The institution of oral anticoagulant therapy requires careful monitoring because of the wide variability in post-operative warfarin response and potential danger of excessive anticoagulation. Higher initial doses, 5 mg or more, frequently cause INR values above the target range. Accordingly, 2.5 mg may be preferable in this particular setting.[23] Following hospital discharge, a structured means for close

TABLE 15.3 — ANTITHROMBOTIC THERAPY FOR PATIENTS WITH NATIVE VALVULAR HEART DISEASE

Native Valvular Heart Disease	Recommendations
Rheumatic Mitral Valvular Disease	
Prior thromboembolism	Oral anticoagulant, INR 2.5
Paroxysmal or chronic AF	Oral anticoagulant, INR 2.5
LA diameter >5.5 cm	Oral anticoagulant, INR 2.5
MVA <1.0 cm^2, LA enlargement (>5.5 cm)	Oral anticoagulant, INR 2.5
Recurrent embolism (despite oral anticoagulant)	Add aspirin (80 to 100 mg qd) or clopidogrel (75 mg qd)
Mitral Annular Calcification	
Uncomplicated	No antithrombotic therapy
AF or systemic embolism	Oral anticoagulant, INR 2.5

Mitral Valve Prolapse	
Uncomplicated	No antithrombotic therapy
TIA	Aspirin (325 mg qd)
Recurrent TIAs	Oral anticoagulant, INR 2.5 or clopidogrel (75 mg qd)
Systemic embolism	Oral anticoagulant, INR 2.5
Aortic Valvular Disease	
Sinus rhythm	No antithrombotic therapy
Chronic AF or systemic embolism	Oral anticoagulant, INR 2.5
Abbreviations: AF, atrial fibrillation; INR, international normalized ratio; LA, left atrium; MVA, mitral valve area; TIA, transient ischemic attack.	

15

TABLE 15.4 — ANTITHROMBOTIC THERAPY FOR PATIENTS WITH BIOPROSTHETIC HEART VALVES OR VALVE REPAIR

Valve Type/Position	INR	Duration of Treatment
Mitral position	2.5	3 months
Aortic position	2.5	3 months
Atrial fibrillation	2.5	Long-term
LA thrombosis	2.5	3 to 6 months
Systemic embolism	2.5	3 to 12 months
Systemic embolism despite anticoagulant therapy	2.5*	Minimum 12 months
Valve repair†	2.5	3 months

Abbreviations: INR, international normalized ratio; LA, left atrium (includes left atrial appendage).

* Add aspirin (80 to 100 mg qd) or clopidogrel (75 mg qd).
† With or without annuloplasty ring.

patient follow-up (coordinated anticoagulation clinic) is recommended.

Summary

Antithrombotic therapy in the form of oral anticoagulation with or without concomitant platelet antagonists is an important consideration for patients with prosthetic as well as those with native valvular heart disease. Each patient should be assessed carefully to determine the inherent risk of thromboembolism, the expected benefit from antithrombotic treatment, and the potential hemorrhagic risk. The development of patient management guidelines and coordinated anticoagulation clinics has streamlined the decision-making process substantially and elevated the standard of care.

TABLE 15.5 — SUMMARY OF RECOMMENDATIONS FOR PATIENTS WITH MECHANICAL HEART VALVES

Valve Type/Position	INR Target
Bileaflet, aortic	2.5 (3.0 if AF, LA >5.5 cm, or LVEF <35%)
Tilting disk, aortic	3.0
Bileaflet, mitral	3.0 or 2.5 plus aspirin 80 to 100 mg qd
Tilting disk, mitral	3.0 or 3.0* plus aspirin 80 to 100 mg qd
Caged-ball/disk	3.0 plus aspirin (80 to 100 mg qd)
Systemic embolism despite anticoagulant therapy	3.0 plus aspirin (80 to 100 mg qd)

Abbreviations: AF, atrial fibrillation; INR, international normalized ratio; LA, left atrium; LVEF, left ventricular ejection fraction.

* With additional risk factors.

REFERENCES

1. Hewson W. Experimental inquiries. I. An inquiry into the properties of the blood, with some remarks on some of its morbid appearances; and an appendix relating to the discovery of the lymphatic system in birds, fish, and the animals called amphibians. London, T Cadell, 1771. Quoted by Wessler S: Thrombosis in the presence of vascular stasis. *Am J Med*. 1962;33:648.

2. Wessler S. Thrombosis in the presence of vascular stasis. *Am J Med*. 1962;33:648.

3. Malone PC, Morris CJ. The sequestration and margination of platelets and leukocytes in veins during conditions of hypokinetic and anaemic hypoxia: potential significance in clinical postoperative venous thrombosis. *J Pathol*. 1978;125:119-129.

4. Sevitt S. The structure and growth of valve-pocket thrombi in femoral veins. *J Clin Pathol*. 1974;27:517-528.

5. Wessler S, Freiman DG, Balloon JD, et al. Experimental pulmonary embolism with serum induced thrombi. *Am J Pathol*. 1961;38:89.

15

6. Scott GB. A quantitative study of the fate of occlusive red venous thrombi. *Br J Exp Pathol.* 1968;49:544-550.

7. Harker LA, Slichter SJ, Sauvage LR. Platelet consumption by arterial prostheses: the effects of endothelialization and pharmacologic inhibition of platelet function. *Ann Surg.* 1977;186;594-601.

8. Clagett GP, Robinowitz M, Maddox Y, Langloss JM, Ramwell PW. The antithrombotic nature of vascular prosthetic pseudointima. *Surgery.* 1982;91:87-94.

9. Cohn LH, Mudge GH, Pratter F, Collins JJ. Five to eight-year follow-up of patients undergoing porcine heart-valve replacement. *N Engl J Med.* 1981;304:258-262.

10. Geha AS, Hammond GL, Laks H, Stansel HC, Glenn WW. Factors affecting performance and thromboembolism after porcine xenograft cardiac valve replacement. *J Thorac Cardiovasc Surg.* 1982;83:377-384.

11. Edmunds LH Jr. Thromboembolic complications of current cardiac valvular prostheses. *Ann Thorac Surg.* 1982;34:96-106.

12. Starr A, Grunkemeier GL. Selection of a prosthetic heart valve. *JAMA.* 1984;251:1739-1742.

13. Yoganathan AP, Corcoran WH, Harrison EC, Carl JR. The Björk-Shiley aortic prosthesis: flow characteristics, thrombus formation and tissue overgrowth. *Circulation.* 1978;58:70-76.

14. Daenen W, Nevelsteen A, van Cauwelaert P, de Maesschalk E, Willems J, Stalpaert G. Nine years' experience with the Björk-Shiley prosthetic valve: early and late results of 932 valve replacements. *Ann Thorac Surg.* 1983;35:651-663.

15. Horstkotte D, Schulte HD, Bircks W, Strauer BE. Lower intensity anticoagulation therapy results in lower complication rates with the St. Jude medical prosthesis. *J Thorac Cardiovasc Surg.* 1994;107: 1136-1145.

16. Vogt S, Hoffmann A, Roth J, et al. Heart valve replacement with the Björk-Shiley and St. Jude medical prostheses: a randomized comparison in 178 patients. *Eur Heart J.* 1990;11:583-591.

17. Acar J, Iung B, Boissel JP, et al. AREVA: multicenter randomized comparison of low-dose versus standard dose anticoagulation in patients with mechanical prosthetic heart valves. *Circulation.* 1996; 94:2107-2112.

18. Sethia B, Turner MA, Lewis S, Rodger RA, Bain WH. Fourteen years' experience with the Björk-Shiley tilting disc prosthesis. *J Thorac Cardiovasc Surg.* 1986;91:350-361.

19. Heras M, Chesebro JH, Fuster V, et al. High risk of thromboemboli early after bioprosthetic cardiac valve replacement. *J Am Coll Cardiol*. 1995;25:1111-1119.

20. Bloomfield P, Kitchin AH, Wheatley DJ, Walbaum PR, Lutz W, Miller HC. A prospective evaluation of the Björk-Shiley, Hancock, and Carpentier-Edwards heart valve prostheses. *Circulation*. 1986;73:1213-1222.

21. Horstkotte D, Piper C, Wiemer M. Optimal frequency of patient monitoring and intensity of oral anticoagulation therapy in valvular heart disease. *J Thromb Thrombolysis*. 1998;5:S19-S24.

22. Sixth ACCP Conference on Antithrombotic Therapy. *Chest*. 2001;119(suppl):1S-370S.

23. Ageno W, Turpie AG, Steidl L, et al. Comparison of a daily fixed 2.5-mg warfarin dose with a 5-mg, international normalized ratio adjusted, warfarin dose initially following heart valve replacement. *Am J Cardiol*. 2001;88:40-44.

15

16   Atrial Fibrillation

Prevalence and Classification

Atrial fibrillation (AF) is a common arrhythmias encountered in routine clinical practice and is an important and independent risk factor for stroke. More than 2 million adults in the United States are afflicted with AF and its prevalence increases markedly with advancing age. AF affects 4% of the population over age 60 and more than 10% of those over 80. AF is more common in men than in women, but since women outnumber men in the older age groups, the total number of men and women with AF is essentially equal.[1]

Patients with AF fall into three categories:
- Valvular or rheumatic
- Nonvalvular
- "Lone."

The prevalence of rheumatic heart disease has decreased dramatically in the past century. Nonvalvular AF is the most common form encountered in clinical practice in North America, often in association with other cardiac conditions such as hypertensive heart disease, heart failure due to systolic or diastolic abnormalities of the left ventricle, and chronic ischemic heart disease. If the absence of organic heart disease, AF is considered "lone."[2]

Risk of Cerebral Thromboembolism

When the left atrium fibrillates, there is stasis of blood flow and increasing likelihood of thrombus formation. Upon release or "embolization" into the circulation, stroke and its attendant disability can occur.

Atrial fibrillation accompanying rheumatic valvular heart disease or a prosthetic valve is associated with a particularly high rate of cerebral thromboembolism. While nonvalvular AF was once considered a harmless disorder, it is now recognized as the most common cause of cardioembolic stroke (Figures 16.1 and 16.2).[3,4]

Although patients with nonvalvular AF are at significant risk for stroke, there are several well recognized risk factors that increase occurrence rates further. These include prior transient ischemic attacks (TIAs) or stroke, history of hypertension, diabetes mellitus, congestive heart failure, angina, and increasing age[1,5] (Table 16.1).

Echocardiography, a diagnostic test that can detect chamber enlargement, valvular regurgitation, and other cardiac abnormalities, can provide important information that guides assessment of stroke risk (Table 16.2).[6,7]

Left atrial enlargement has been suggested as a risk factor for stroke, although its positive predictive value remains unproven.[6] The left atrium and its appendage are well visualized by transesophageal echocardiography (TEE) because of the close proximity of the left atrium to the esophagus. The appearance of spontaneous echo contrast "or smoke" in the left atrium suggests stasis of blood flow and, with it, a greater risk for thrombosis in the left atrium or its appendage. The presence of left atrial thrombus substantially increases the risk for thromboembolism.[6-8]

Effectiveness of Antithrombotic Therapy

The goals for the clinical management of AF are to 1) determine, and whenever possible, correct the underlying pro-arrhythmic substrate, and 2) reduce the adverse hemodynamic and thromboembolic consequences of the arrhythmia through control of ventricular rate and maintenance of sinus rhythm. Because normal sinus rhythm may not be achieved or sustained easily, the focus of attention often shifts to stroke prevention by means of antithrombotic therapy. Although a majority of patients with AF are candidates for anticoagulation therapy, a relatively small proportion actually receive it.[9] In both community and academic settings, fewer than half of patients with strong indications for anticoagulation therapy are actually prescribed warfarin.[10,11]

FIGURE 16.1 — STROKE: EMBOLI OF CARDIAC ORIGIN

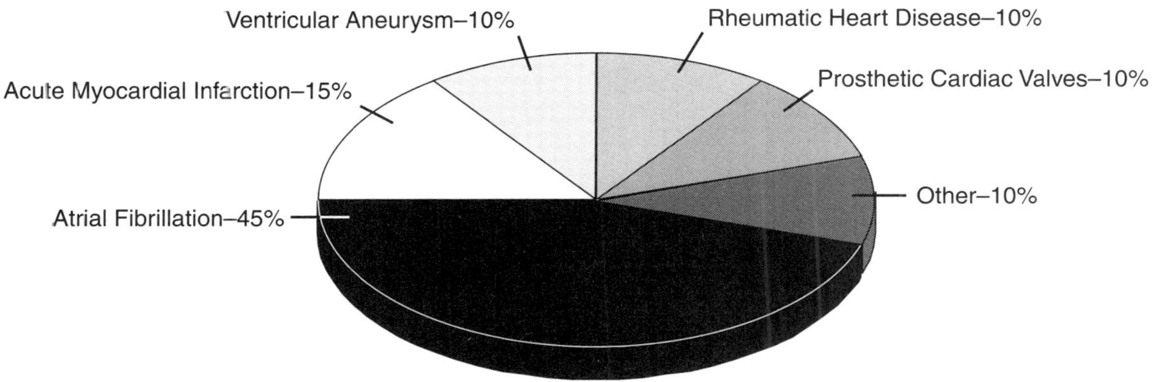

Atrial fibrillation is the most common condition that can cause intracardiac thrombi and embolization of thrombotic material, accounting for nearly half of all emboli of cardiac origin.

Cerebral Embolism Task Force. *Arch Neurol.* 1986;43:71-84.

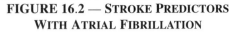

FIGURE 16.2 — STROKE PREDICTORS WITH ATRIAL FIBRILLATION

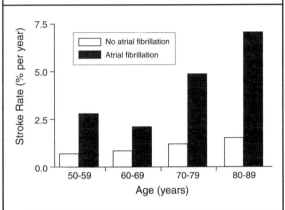

Stroke incidence increases with age for the general population; however, the overall incidence is particularly high in aging adults with atrial fibrillation.

Wolf PA, et al. *Neurology*. 1978;28:973-977.

Five large-scale randomized clinical trials performed in Denmark, the United States, and Canada[12,13,16-18] have shown definitively that oral anticoagulation therapy with warfarin, titrated to an international normalized ratio (INR) of 2.0 to 4.5 prevents stroke with a very low risk for major hemorrhage (Table 16.3).

A meta-analysis of randomized trials demonstrated that anticoagulation therapy reduced the risk of stroke by 68%, with almost no increase in the frequency of intracranial or major bleeding.[5] Women experienced an even greater reduction in stroke risk (84%) compared with men (60%).[5] Based on the existence of strong and compelling data, an expert panel of the American College of Chest Physicians issued a directive for the use of anticoagulation therapy with warfarin in appropriately chosen patients with AF.[1] According to their consensus recommendations, oral warfarin therapy titrated to a goal INR of 2.5, range 2 to 3, should be strongly considered for all eligible patients who are at high risk for stroke.[1]

TABLE 16.1 — STROKE PREDICTORS WITH ATRIAL FIBRILLATION: RISK-STRATIFICATION SCHEME

Stratification	Clinical Features	Stroke Rate (%/y)
High risk	Prior stroke or TIA or systemic embolism; age >75, hypertension, poor LV systolic function; rheumatic mitral valve disease or prosthetic heart valve	4 to 12
Moderate risk	Age 65 to 75; CAD with preserved LV function, thyrotoxicosis	2 to 4
Low risk	No high- or moderate-risk features, eg <65 years old, and no cardiovascular disease	1

Abbreviations: CAD, coronary artery disease; LV, left ventricular; TIA, transient ischemic attack.

Fintel D, Hofmann C. *The American Family Physicians Guide to Preventing Strokes and Lowering Health Risks in Patients With Atrial Fibrillation.* Lisle, Ill: Illinois Academy of Family Physicians; 2000; and Albers G, et al. *Chest.* 2001;119:194S-206S.

Risk Stratification and Risk Reduction With Warfarin Therapy

Risk stratification can be used to reliably identify patients who are at high risk for stroke and those who will benefit most from anticoagulation therapy. Treatment reduces absolute stroke rates by 3.2%, 4.0%, and 6.9% for patients with AF and concomitant risk factors who are <65, 65 to 75, and >75 years of age, respectively.[5] Thus warfarin therapy in older patients with AF can result in a substantial reduction (70% to 85% relative risk) for life-threatening and crippling consequences of stroke. Even in the un-

16

TABLE 16.2 — STROKE PREDICTORS WITH ATRIAL FIBRILLATION: ECHOCARDIOGRAPHIC FINDINGS

Transthoracic Echo (TTE)
- Left ventricular ejection fraction <50%
- Large left atrium (>2.5 cm/M^2 body surface area)

Transesophageal Echo (TEE)
- Echo "smoke" in left atrium
- Left atrial appendage thrombus

Fintel D, Hofmann C. *The American Family Physicians Guide to Preventing Strokes and Lowering Health Risks in Patients With Atrial Fibrillation.* Lisle, Ill: Illinois Academy of Family Physicians; 2000.

TABLE 16.3 — STROKE REDUCTION BY WARFARIN THERAPY

Warfarin reduced the risk of stroke by:
- 68% overall
- 60% in men
- 84% in women

Atrial Fibrillation Investigators. *Arch Intern Med.* 1994;154:1449-1457.

common circumstance of elderly patients (>75 years) with no other risk factors, treatment with warfarin can reduce the risk of stroke considerably.[1]

The epidemiology-based concept of "number needed to treat to show benefit" is useful in understanding the impact of anticoagulation therapy; combining the absolute rate of stroke with the relative reduction in stroke risk provided by warfarin therapy (Table 16.4).[2,20] The data demonstrate that only 15 patients with prior stroke or TIA would require warfarin treatment for 1 year to prevent a life-threatening or disabling stroke. The higher the clinical risk of stroke, the greater the protection afforded by anticoagulation. When more than one risk factor is present, increased age strikingly decreases the "number needed to treat," clearly demonstrating the elevated stroke risk in older patients with additional risk factors.

TABLE 16.4 — NUMBER OF ATRIAL FIBRILLATION PATIENTS TREATED WITH WARFARIN TO PREVENT A STROKE

Category	Actual Risk Reduction Rate (%/y)	Number Needed to Treat
Age <65 years and one or more risk factors	3.2	31
Age 65 to 75 years, and one or more risk factors	4.0	25
Age >75 years, and one or more risk factors	6.9	14
Hypertension	3.7	27
Diabetes	5.8	17
Prior stroke or transient ischemic attack	6.6	15
Congestive heart failure	5.2	19
Angina pectoris	5.8	17
Myocardial infarction	4.9	20

Fintel D, Hofmann C. *The American Family Physicians Guide to Preventing Strokes and Lowering Health Risks in Patients With Atrial Fibrillation.* Lisle, Ill: Illinois Academy of Family Physicians; 2000.

16

Risks Versus Benefits of Warfarin Therapy

The major risk of anticoagulation therapy is bleeding, particularly in the presence of gastrointestinal or genitourinary disease, or in a setting where trauma is more likely (alcoholism, Parkinson's disease, or previous stroke with significant neurologic impairment). However, despite the potential for increased bleeding risk, pooled data from the five largest randomized trials of anticoagulation therapy demonstrate only a small increase in risk for major hemorrhage in patients treated with warfarin compared with control groups—1% vs 1.3% annually (Table 16.5, Figure 16.3).[5]

The Role of Antiplatelet Agents

Thrombus developing within the left atrium or left atrial appendage in atrial fibrillation is dependent upon stasis of blood flow (and activation of soluble coagulation factors); however, several studies have evaluated the reduction of stroke risk by aspirin therapy, administered in doses of 75 mg to 325 mg.[12-14] In two randomized trials, Danish Atrial Fibrillation Aspirin Coagulation (AFASAK)[12] and European Atrial Fibrillation Trial (EAFT),[14] risk reduction with aspirin failed to achieve statistical significance (16% and 17%, respectively). In contrast, the American Stroke Prevention in Atrial Fibrillation (SPAF)-1 trial,[13] showed a significant reduction (42%) with aspirin treatment. A pooled analysis of these three trials demonstrated a 21% reduction in the risk of ischemic stroke (8.1% in control patients and 6.3% in aspirin-treated patients; $P = 0.05$; number needed to treat = 50).[1,21] Suggesting that aspirin therapy is associated with a clinically important decrease in stroke risk among patients with AF. Several studies directly compared the efficacy of aspirin with warfarin. In the AFASAK[12] and EAFT[14] trials, warfarin therapy significantly decreased the risk of primary events by 48% and 40%, respectively, as compared with aspirin. The SPAF-3 study evaluated the efficacy of fixed-dose, low-intensity warfarin therapy (INR 1.2 to 1.5; maximum daily dose, 3 mg) plus aspirin.[15] This

TABLE 16.5 — RISK OF BLEEDING: ANNUAL OCCURRENCE OF MAJOR BLEEDING EVENTS

Event	Frequency (%)
Major Bleeding	
Patients receiving placebo	1.0
Warfarin-treated patients	1.3
Intracranial Bleeding	
Patients receiving placebo	0.1
Warfarin-treated patients	0.3

Atrial Fibrillation Investigators. *Arch Intern Med* 1994;154:1449-1457.

arm was prematurely terminated because of a substantially increased rate of primary outcome events (7.9% per year) compared with patients receiving standard adjusted-dose warfarin, target INR 2 to 3 (1.9% per year). All patients participating in this trial had at least one clinical risk factor for stroke. Thus low-intensity anticoagulation plus aspirin is ineffective in high-risk patients.[15] In addition, there is a considerably greater risk reduction associated with warfarin therapy (68%) than with aspirin therapy (21%) in high-risk patients when compared with control patients.[5] Considered collectively, the data support aspirin treatment solely for patients at low risk for stroke (<65 years old and no other risk factors) or those who have contraindications for warfarin therapy.[2]

Clopidogrel and ticlopidine are effective for stroke prevention, however, there are no clinical trial data supporting their primary use in patients with AF

Initiating and Monitoring Antithrombotic Therapy

The initial evaluation of a patient with AF should include a careful history, physical examination, selected laboratory studies, and diagnostic tests as indicated[2] (Table 16.6). Table 16.7 displays recommendations for warfarin or aspi-

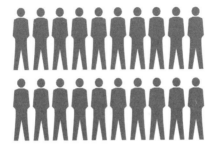

rin therapy, dependent on age and the presence or absence of other risk factors.[1, 2]

When initiating outpatient warfarin therapy in the outpatient setting, clinicians must be mindful of differing dose requirements and potential interactions (Figure 16.4). Initial starting doses are typically 5 mg in patients under 65 years of age, decreasing to 3 mg in patients over 75. Since warfarin exerts its action by preventing hepatic carboxylation of vitamin K–dependent clotting factors, 3 to 5 days

TABLE 16.6 — RECOMMENDED STRATEGY FOR MANAGING PATIENTS WITH ATRIAL FIBRILLATION

- Slow ventricular response
- Identify and correct the underlying triggers/causes of AF
- Assess risks vs benefits of electrical or pharmacologic cardioversion. Before and after cardioversion, use anticoagulant therapy according to ACCP guidelines
- For a patient who remains in chronic or paroxysmal AF, anticoagulate with warfarin (target INR 2.5, range 2 to 3). Aspirin therapy is recommended for patients < 65 with "lone AF"

Abbreviations: AF, atrial fibrillation; ACCP, American College of Chest Physicians; INR, international normalized ratio.

TABLE 16.7 — CHEST 2001 SUMMARY OF RECOMMENDATIONS

Age (y)	Risk Factors*	Recommendation
<65	Absent	Aspirin
	Present	Warfarin (target INR 2.5, range 2 to 3)
65-75	Absent	Aspirin or warfarin
	Present	Warfarin (target INR 2.5, range 2 to 3)
>75	All patients	Warfarin (target INR 2.5, range 2 to 3)

Abbreviation: INR, international normalized ratio.

* Prior transient ischemic attack, systemic embolus or stroke, hypertension, poor left ventricular function, rheumatic mitral valve disease, prosthetic heart valve.

Albers G, et al. *Chest.* 2001;119:194S-206S.

16

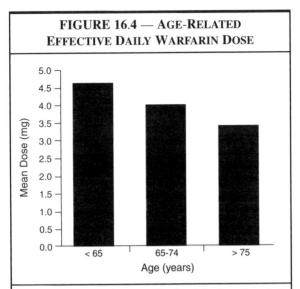

FIGURE 16.4 — AGE-RELATED EFFECTIVE DAILY WARFARIN DOSE

With increasing age, the mean effective daily dose of warfarin diminishes.

are generally required to achieve a full anticoagulation effect. Given delayed expression of drug effect, along with the increased sensitivity of older individuals to warfarin, it is appropriate to "go low and slow" when initiating therapy and to change weekly dose by only 1 to 2 mg at a time when INR values fall out of the therapeutic range of 2 to 3. When initiating therapy, anticoagulation status should be monitored every 1 to 3 days until the INR is stable, followed by weekly monitoring. Routine monthly testing is appropriate once patients have stabilized. An INR should be checked within 3 days of starting or stopping medications known to interact with warfarin and at any time the patient experiences signs or symptoms of bleeding or thrombosis.[2]

The therapeutic window is the level of therapy that achieves an optimal balance between patient benefit and risk. When administering anticoagulation therapy for AF, this window is the range of anticoagulation intensity, measured by the INR, which reliably prevents thromboembolic events with a minimum risk of hemorrhagic events. Hylek et al[24] based on a large anticoagulation clinic population, reported that the risk of thromboembolic events in patients with AF rises dramatically with an INR <2, doubling at an INR of 1.7, and tripling at an INR of 1.5 (Figure 16.5). Conversely, the risk of hemorrhage increases dramatically as the INR increases to levels >3 (Figure 16.6).[25] The therapeutic window (Figure 16.7) therefore represents the optimum INR range of 2 to 3, at which the risks of both hemorrhage and thromboemboli are minimized.

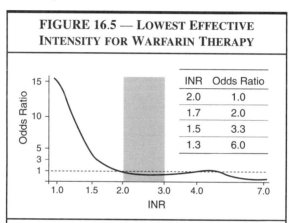

FIGURE 16.5 — LOWEST EFFECTIVE INTENSITY FOR WARFARIN THERAPY

INR	Odds Ratio
2.0	1.0
1.7	2.0
1.5	3.3
1.3	6.0

Hylek and colleagues studied the lowest effective intensity for anticoagulant therapy with warfarin. They determined that an intensity of anticoagulation expressed as international normalized ratio (INR) values below 2.0 resulted in a substantially higher risk of stroke.

Hylek EM, et al. *N Engl J Med.* 1996;335:540-546.

Improving the Paradigm for Outpatient Anticoagulation

The traditional approach to outpatient anticoagulation therapy management involves phlebotomy, a delay period (to receive test results from an outside laboratory), retrieval of the patient's records, attempts by the office staff (nurse or physician) to reach the patient and discuss changes in dose, and documentation of these changes in the medical record. The development of rapid and reliable point-of-care coagulation monitors, such as the CoaguChek and ProTime

16

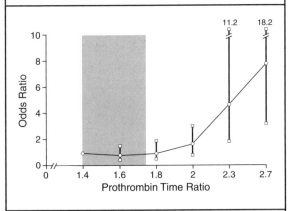

FIGURE 16.6 — RISK OF INTRACRANIAL HEMORRHAGE (OUTPATIENTS)

This graph displays the risk of intracranial hemorrhage in outpatients treated with warfarin. A prothrombin time ratio (PTR) >2.0, roughly corresponding to an international normalized ratio (INR) of 3.7 to 4.3 resulted in an increase in the risk of bleeding. The estimated odds ratio of subdural hemorrhage increased 7.6-fold as the PTR increased from 2.0 to 2.5. Note: Shade to PTR = 1.75.

Hylek EM, Singer DE. *Ann Intern Med*. 1994;120:897-902.

devices, offers an attractive alternative. This technology, coupled with computerized data bases and experienced anticoagulation clinic providers represents an emerging coordinated strategy to achieve optimal care. Anticoagulation clinics, whether based in the hospital or in an outpatient-practice setting, have demonstrated clear benefits over a traditional office-based approach, including reduced episodes of under- or over-anticoagulation, clinical events, hospitalizations, and emergency room (ER) visits (Table 16.8).[27]

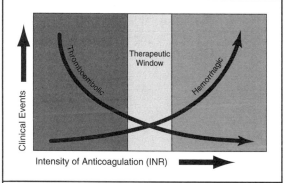

FIGURE 16.7 — THERAPEUTIC WINDOW

Thromboembolic events may occur at an international normalized ratio (INR) value of less than 2.0. Conversely, clinical events associated with hemorrhage increase with increasing intensity of anticoagulation. The Chest 2001 Guidelines recommend a target INR of 2.5 (range 2.0 to 3.0) for atrial fibrillation.

Challenges for the Future: Improving the Delivery of Antithrombotic Therapy for Atrial Fibrillation

The utilization of warfarin and aspirin therapy for stroke prevention in AF has increased substantially in the past decade,[28] due in part to the publication of landmark trials demonstrating the benefit of treatment and the promulgation of guidelines by the Consensus Committee of the American College of Chest Physicians. Recent trends suggest, however, that treatment rates have plateaued — a concerning trend which mandates national education efforts for physicians and health care systems regarding treatment choices in patients with AF (Figure 16.8). The implementation of anticoagulation therapy with warfarin could prevent 40,000 strokes per year, at a cost saving of more than $600 million annually.[9]

TABLE 16.8 — MONITORING ANTICOAGULATION OUTCOMES: ANTICOAGULATION CLINICS VS USUAL MEDICAL CARE

Anticoagulation Outcome	Clinics (%)	Usual (%)
Rates of bleeding	8.1	35.3
Rates of thromboembolic events	3.3	11.8
Incidence of warfarin-related:		
Hospitalizations	5.0	19.0
Emergency-room visits	6.0	22.0

Chiquette E, et al. *Arch Intern Med.* 1998;158:1641-1647.

FIGURE 16.8 — WARFARIN UTILIZATION

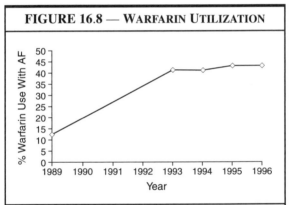

When evaluating warfarin use in 2.8 million patient visits over an 8-year period, it is obvious that warfarin use increased after the publication of results of several randomized clinical trials that evaluated stroke prevention in atrial fibrillation (AF). Subsequent utilization has remained constant (flat) despite additional publications on the efficacy of warfarin in stroke prevention and the underutilization of antithrombotic therapy in patients with AF.

Stafford RS, Singer DE. *Circulation.* 1998;97:1231-1233.

Summary

Atrial fibrillation is a common arrhythmia with a prevalence that increases with age. Patients with AF have an increased risk for thromboembolic complications, most importantly, stroke. The results of several international large-scale, randomized trials have provided convincing evidence that coexisting demographic and clinical characteristics determine the overall likelihood of stroke. Furthermore, these studies demonstrate conclusively that antithrombotic therapy with warfarin in patients at moderate or high risk and with aspirin in patients at low risk or those unable or unwilling to take warfarin, can significantly reduce thromboembolic complications, with enormous potential savings in human suffering and economic cost. Comprehensive approaches to management that include point of care coagulation monitoring and coordinating anticoagulation clinics offer great promise in elevating the standard of care.

REFERENCES

1. Albers G, Dalen J, Laupacis A, et al. Antithrombotic therapy in atrial fibrillation. *Chest.* 2001;199:194S-206S.

2. Fintel D, Hofmann C. *The American Family Physicians Guide to Preventing Strokes and Lowering Health Risks in Patients With Atrial Fibrillation.* Lisle, Ill: Illinois Academy of Family Physicians; 2000.

3. Cerebral Embolism Task Force. Cardiogenic brain embolism. *Arch Neurol.* 1986;43:71-84.

4. Wolf PA, Dawber TR, Thomas HE Jr, Kannel WB. Epidemiologic assessment of chronic atrial fibrillation and risk of stroke: the Framingham Study. *Neurology.* 1978;28:973-977.

5. Atrial Fibrillation Investigators. Risk factors for stroke and efficacy of antithrombotic therapy in atrial fibrillation. Analysis of pooled data from five randomized controlled trials [published correction appears in *Arch Intern Med.* 1994;154:2254]. *Arch Intern Med.* 1994;154:1449-1457.

6. Atrial Fibrillation Investigators. Echocardiographic predictors of stroke in patients with atrial fibrillation: a prospective study of 1066 patients from 3 clinical trials. *Arch Intern Med.* 1998;158:1316-1320.

7. Ezekowitz MD, Levine JA. Preventing stroke in patients with atrial fibrillation. *JAMA.* 1999;281:1830-1835.

16

8. Stroke Prevention in Atrial Fibrillation Investigators Committee on Echocardiography. Transesophageal echocardiographic correlates of thromboembolism in high-risk patients with nonvalvular atrial fibrillation. *Ann Intern Med.* 1987;147:1561-1564.

9. Patient Outcomes Research Team. Secondary and tertiary prevention of stroke. Agency for Health Care Policy and Research (AHCPR); 1995. Publication 95-0091.

10. Stafford RS, Singer DE. Recent national patterns of warfarin use in atrial fibrillation. *Circulation.* 1998;97:1231-1233.

11. Brass LM, Krumholz HM, Scinto JD, Mathur D, Radford M. Warfarin use following ischemic stroke among Medicare patients with atrial fibrillation. *Arch Intern Med.* 1998;158:2093-2100.

12. Peterson P, Boysen G, Godtfredsen J, Anderson ED, Anderson B. Placebo controlled randomised trial of warfarin and aspirin for prevention of thromboembolic complications in chronic atrial fibrillation. The Copenhagen AFASAK study. *Lancet.* 1989;1:175-179.

13. Stroke Prevention in Atrial Fibrillation Investigators. Stroke Prevention in Atrial Fibrillation Study. Final results. *Circulation.* 1991;84: 527-539.

14. European Atrial Fibrillation Trial Study Group. Optimal oral anticoagulation therapy in patients with nonrheumatic atrial fibrillation and recent cerebral ischemia. *N Engl J Med.* 1995;333:5-10.

15. Stroke Prevention in Atrial Fibrillation Investigators. Adjusted-dose warfarin versus low-intensity, fixed-dose warfarin plus aspirin for high-risk patients with atrial fibrillation: stroke prevention in atrial fibrillation III randomized clinical trial. *Lancet.* 1996;348:633-638.

16. Boston Area Anticoagulation Trial for Atrial Fibrillation Investigators. The effect of low-dose warfarin on the risk of stroke in patients with nonrheumatic atrial fibrillation. *N Engl J Med.* 1990;323:1505-1511.

17. Connolly SJ, Laupacis A, Gent M, Roberts RS, Cairns JA, Joyner C. Canadian Atrial Fibrillation Anticoagulation (CAFA) Study. *J Am Coll Cardiol.* 1991;18:349-355.

18. Ezekowitz MD, Bridgers SL, James KE, et al for the Veterans Affairs Stroke Prevention in Nonrheumatic Atrial Fibrillation Investigators. Warfarin in the prevention of stroke associated with nonrheumatic atrial fibrillation. *N Engl J Med.* 1992;327:1406-1412.

19. Anand SS, Yusuf S. Oral anticoagulant therapy in patients with coronary artery disease: a meta-analysis. *JAMA.* 1999;282:2058-2067.

20. Akhtar W, Reeves WE, Movahed A. Indications for anticoagulation in atrial fibrillation [published correction appears in *Am Fam Physician.* 1999;59:1122]. *Am Fam Physician.* 1998;58:130-136.

21. Fihn S, Callahan CM, Martin DC, McDonnell MB, Henikoff JG, White RH. The risk for and severity of bleeding complications in elderly patients treated with warfarin. The National Consortium of Anticoagulation Clinics. *Ann Intern Med*. 1996;124:970-979.

22. Gladman JR, Dolan G. Effect of age upon the induction and maintenance of anticoagulation with warfarin. *Postgrad Med J*. 1995;71: 153-155.

23. Lieberman R, Nelson R. Dose-response and concentration-response relationships: clinical and regulatory perspectives. *Ther Drug Monit*. 1993;15:498-502.

24. Hylek EM, Skates SJ, Sheehan MA, Singer DE. An analysis of the lowest effective intensity of prophylactic anticoagulation for patients with nonrheumatic atrial fibrillation. *N Engl J Med*. 1996;335:540-545.

25. Hylek EM, Singer DE. Risk factors for intracranial hemorrhage in outpatients taking warfarin. *Ann Intern Med*. 1994;120:897-902.

26. CoumaCare. Wilmington, Del: Du Pont Pharma; 1997.

27. Chiquette E, Amato MG, Bussey HI, et al. Comparison of an anticoagulation clinic with usual medical care: anticoagulation control, patient outcomes, and health care costs. *Arch Intern Med*. 1998;158: 1641-1647.

28. Stafford RS, Singer DE. Recent national patterns of warfarin use in atrial fibrillation. *Circulation*. 1998;97:1231-1233.

16

17 Venous Thromboembolic Disease and Pulmonary Embolism

Incidence

Venous thromboembolism is common and leads to disability, economic loss, and even death. The true incidence is uncertain, but a report from Minnesota provides some revealing statistics.[1] The health records of 2218 persons residing in Olmstead County over a 25-year period having a deep vein thrombosis (DVT) or pulmonary embolism (PE) were reviewed. The rate of DVT was 48 per 100,000, and PE, 69 per 100,000. Projected to the entire US population, this would be 201,000 new cases of venous thromboembolism per year (107,000 DVT and 94,000 PE).

Anatomy and Pathophysiology

The venous anatomy of the lower extremities is complex and varies from person to person.[2] Constant features are the proximal veins: the iliacs, common femoral, superficial and deep femoral, and popliteals (Figure 17.1). The iliac veins are in the pelvis and the common femoral is a very short segment extending under the inguinal ligament. The superficial femoral vein is the major, long conduit down the thigh to the knee. The deep femoral vein is rarely the site of disease. The popliteal vein branches into the anterior and posterior tibial veins and the peroneal vein in highly variable fashion. These veins distal to the popliteal vein are the major calf veins; there are also soleal and gastrocnemius veins. The greater and lesser saphenous veins are the superficial veins of the leg, and connect to the deep system via perforating veins. Patients may have a superficial thrombophlebitis (reported to occur frequently in patients with Factor V Leiden), calf vein thrombosis, proximal vein thrombosis, or various combinations of proximal and distal vein clots.

17

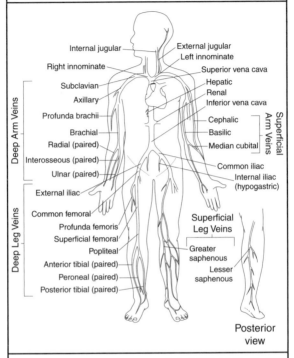

FIGURE 17.1 — GROSS ANATOMY OF THE SYSTEMIC VENOUS SYSTEM

Fahey VA (ed). In: *Vascular Nursing*, 3rd ed. Philadelphia, Pa: WB Saunders Co; 1999:23.

More than 100 years ago, Virchow established that thrombi forming in the veins of the lower extremities or pelvis could embolize to the lungs.[3] He described his famous triad of risk factors for venous thromboembolism:

- Blood hypercoagulability
- Stasis of flow
- Vessel-wall injury.

The factors that have been associated with hypercoagulability may be congenital, acquired, or both, and are discussed in Chapter 11, *Inherited/Acquired Coagulation and Platelet Disorders (Thrombophilia)*. However, it must be emphasized that it is a combination of risk factors that most often is associated with venous thrombosis. It is unlikely that only two or three risk factors are involved in the actual development of a thrombus; for example, a study that recorded simply whether patients were heterozygous for Factor V Leiden preoperatively did not find an association with the postoperative development of thromboembolism after joint arthroplasty.[4] As more reliable associations are made between risk factors and venous thrombosis, screening for multiple risk factors prior to surgery or pharmacotherapy may become an accepted procedure.

Stewart,[5] in an experimental model of venous thrombosis, describes four stages in the pathogenesis of venous thrombi:

- *Stage 1*: Initiation, characterized by the development of small tears in the endothelium of thin-walled veins.
- *Stage 2*: Adherence of neutrophils and platelets, with release of cathepsin, neutrophil activation peptide-2, β-thromboglobulin, and adenosine diphosphate.
- *Stage 3*: Coagulation, associated with platelet activation and fibrin deposition.
- *Stage 4*: Layering, characterized by trapping of erythrocytes and activation of neutrophils and platelets by fibrin.

Thrombi form within the cusps of venous valves and gradually accrete fibrin (stage 4) until they either obstruct the lumen or embolize. The factors determining which path is followed are obscure. Large thrombi may be found occluding major veins with no evidence of embolization, or massive pulmonary embolization may occur with no apparent residual thrombi in the major veins. In animal studies, Wessler and associates[6] observed that 5 days were required for experimentally formed emboli to become adherent to the subendothelium of the pulmonary arteries. Whether a similar period is necessary for pathologic thrombi to attach to human veins is unknown but might have an important bearing on when activity should be permitted after a DVT is diagnosed.[7]

One reason for difficulty in determining the duration of a thrombosis is that there may be no symptoms as long

17

as the thrombi do not completely occlude the vein lumen. However, such thrombi may embolize at any time; this accounts for the presence of pulmonary emboli in patients who have never had leg symptoms. Furthermore, most noninvasive tests for DVT rely on detection of venous occlusion as a surrogate marker for venous thrombosis. Non-obstructing thrombi are frequently not recognized by these techniques but become apparent on radiocontrast venography (see below).

Diagnosis

The diagnosis of DVT and PE is difficult and requires a mixture of clinical suspicion and objective testing.[8] A complete history, with attention to specific symptoms and signs, should be recorded; a thorough family history is also invaluable. The laboratory evaluation is critical in establishing an unequivocal diagnosis, but most of the tests currently used are not of uniformly high sensitivity and specificity. Thus, an accurate diagnosis requires experience and attention to detail.

Signs and Symptoms of Deep Vein Thrombosis

The cardinal symptoms of DVT are pain and swelling in the lower extremity. The pain may be sharp and sudden in onset or come on more gradually and be reported as drawing in character. There may be little or no swelling, or the entire lower extremity may be enormous. On examination, there is frequently a reddish-purple discoloration of the leg in comparison with the noninvolved side. One may also see a prominent venous pattern on the affected limb. If there is associated superficial phlebitis, there may be tenderness over the saphenous vein itself and a cord may be palpable; otherwise, diffuse calf tenderness, and warmth of the leg may be present. The Homans' sign (pain in the calf with dorsiflexion of the foot) is present in only about half the cases and is neither sensitive nor specific for DVT.

Deep vein thrombosis may be simulated by a ruptured Baker's cyst. These cysts are often located in the popliteal fossa; when they rupture, they produce sudden, severe pain, redness, swelling, and leg tenderness mimicking the signs and symptoms of DVT. Another "look-alike" is a simple cellulitis, which is usually associated with redness of the skin, warmth, swelling, and pain. Heterotopic ossification occurs in the thigh and pelvic girdle muscles of persons with spinal cord injury and motor paralysis. The deposition of calcium salts in the muscles results in redness and warmth of the overlying skin and swelling of the involved muscle groups, simulating proximal vein thrombosis. Large hematomas of the thigh may produce warmth, leg swelling, tenderness, and skin discoloration. Leg pains may be due to muscle cramps, and leg swelling occurs in heart failure and pregnancy, though usually bilaterally. Because there are so many entities that may be confused with DVT, laboratory studies are required to confirm the diagnosis.

Signs and Symptoms of Pulmonary Embolism

Patients with PE may be entirely asymptomatic or complain only of vague fatigue or breathlessness on exertion. Chest pain may be absent or described as a lancinating pain with every breath, making any activity impossible. Occasionally, patients note only a dull ache, a feeling of chest heaviness, or palpitations. Cough and hemoptysis are relatively infrequent. Often, PE is associated with otherwise unexplained fever (with temperature as high as 39°C). Tachycardia is the rule, tachypnea is often present, and if the embolus is large, syncope may occur. Chest examination may be entirely unremarkable, or there may be dullness and decreased breath sounds at one lung base, indicating the presence of a pleural effusion. Infrequently, a pleural rub is present. Sometimes, there is rib tenderness, leading to the mistaken impression that symptoms are due to chest trauma rather than to PE.

17

The differential diagnosis is broad and includes pneumonia, pleurisy, pneumothorax, atelectasis, pulmonary edema, congestive heart failure, bronchitis, lung malignancy, septicemia, orthostasis, and musculoskeletal pain. Even experienced clinicians may mistake one of these disorders for PE. Therefore, objective testing is essential whenever the diagnosis is suspected.

Laboratory Testing for Deep Vein Thrombosis

A diagnostic algorithm has been proposed by Perrier and Bounameaux (Figure 17.2).[9] The first step is the performance of a rapid and sensitive test for d-dimer; several such tests, such as SimpliRed (AGEN® Biomedical, Ltd. Brisbane, Australia) and Vidas DD® (bioMerieux, Marcy l'Etoile, France), have been studied extensively.[10,11] D-dimer is a proteolytic product of the degradation of fibrin, and is released into the circulation when fibrin thrombi undergo lysis. A negative test reliably excludes thrombosis unless there is a moderate or high pre-test probability of thrombosis.[10] Factors that affect pre-test probability are the presence of active cancer, paralysis or lower extremity cast, major surgery within the previous 4 weeks or bedridden for more than 3 days, tenderness along the deep veins, thigh, and/or calf swelling, or a strong family history of venous thromboembolism.[12] If these are present, or if the physician considers that thromboembolism is the most likely explanation for the patient's symptoms based on other findings,[13] then further testing must be performed. Additional testing is also required if the d-dimer is positive, since false positive results may occur in patients with liver or kidney disease, as well as after trauma or surgery. The next step is to perform duplex ultrasound.[14] This noninvasive technique provides a clear diagnosis in the majority of patients with symptomatic thrombi. The veins of greatest interest (common femoral, superficial femoral, popliteal) are readily located; they should be easily compressible by the ultrasound transducer. Lack of compressibility is characteristic of venous thrombosis and indicates venous hypertension due to outflow obstruction by thrombus. Thrombi may occasionally be visualized and collateral circulation recognized. A review of nine published studies[15] noted that the sensitivity and specificity of compression ultrasound in the diagnosis of symptomatic proximal vein thrombosis were 96% and 98%, respectively. In asymptomatic patients, complete

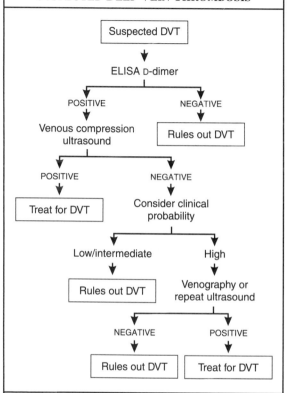

FIGURE 17.2 — DIAGNOSTIC ALGORITHM FOR SUSPECTED DEEP VEIN THROMBOSIS

Suspected DVT

↓

ELISA D-dimer

POSITIVE → Venous compression ultrasound

NEGATIVE → Rules out DVT

Venous compression ultrasound:

POSITIVE → Treat for DVT

NEGATIVE → Consider clinical probability

Low/intermediate → Rules out DVT

High → Venography or repeat ultrasound

NEGATIVE → Rules out DVT

POSITIVE → Treat for DVT

Abbreviations: DVT, deep vein thrombosis; ELISA, enzyme-linked immunosorbent assay.

From: Perrier A, Bounameaux H. *Thromb Haemost.* 2001, 86:475-487.

obstruction of the veins is usually not present, and veins may remain compressible. Under these circumstances, the sensitivity of ultrasound declines to 62%, although the test remains very specific (97%). Sensitivity is also lost in patients with calf-vein thrombosis, where the vagaries of the venous anatomy in the calf may mislead the ultrasonographer, and up to 60% of thrombi may be missed. Other limitations of ultrasound include having only a short segment of vein involved and attempting to recognize fresh thrombus in a patient with old DVT.[14]

When there is strong clinical suspicion of DVT but the ultrasound is negative or equivocal, contrast venography is the test of choice. This is an invasive procedure which entails injecting contrast material into a vein on the dorsum of the foot and using fluoroscopy to follow the course of the dye as it makes its way to the pelvis. If an appropriate amount of contrast is injected, all veins with the exception of the deep femoral vein are visualized.

Diagnostic Testing for Pulmonary Embolism

A diagnostic algorithm for pulmonary embolism is shown in Figure 17.3. Again, one begins with the rapid d-dimer test, which is usually very sensitive to the presence of pulmonary emboli. In a patient with low clinical probability, a negative test rules out pulmonary embolism;[13] if the test is positive, compression ultrasound will indicate whether deep vein thrombosis is present. Identification of a thrombus is an indication for anticoagulant therapy. The ventilation/perfusion lung scan has traditionally been selected as the initial method for the objective diagnosis of PE. Interpretation of the test requires a concomitant chest x-ray, which most often is either normal or shows an effusion. Other signs, such as Hampton's hump or prominent pulmonary vasculature, are far less frequent. The lung scan is performed by doing a ventilation scan using xenon and a perfusion scan with iodinated albumin microspheres. A ventilated area that is not perfused is prima facie evidence of a PE, especially if the chest x-ray is normal in the area of interest. Unfortunately, such positive scans are found in only 15% of cases, and normal scans occur in only 8%; the majority of scans are of intermediate (44%) or low (33%) probability.[16] Thus lung scanning alone is not helpful in a majority of patients. Efforts have been made to improve the diagnostic value of lung scans by combining the scan results with the clinical assessment of disease likelihood.[12] For example, if there is a high clinical probability of a PE and the scan is positive, then a PE can be confirmed by pulmonary angiography 96% of the time. On the other hand, if there is a low clinical probability and the scan is a low-probability scan, PE is present in only 4%. For intermediate scans, the probabilities improve from 50% to 66% with high clinical probability and to 16% with low clinical probability.

Ventilation/perfusion scans are clearly not optimal studies for PE and are being supplanted as first-line tests by helical computerized tomography (CT). This technique displays thrombi located in the main pulmonary arteries. In institutions with the appropriate equipment, helical CT has the advantage that it is available at all times, whereas lung scans are usually obtainable only during regular hours. A disadvantage is lack of sensitivity to smaller emboli. Two critical analyses of the literature concluded that CT has not yet been evaluated by high quality studies.[17,18] One algorithm suggests that CT be performed in all patients in whom there is an intermediate or high clinical suspicion of PE. If no PE is demonstrated, ultrasound of the legs could be done to ensure that thrombi are not present,[15] and anticoagulants would be withheld. This approach needs to be examined in a controlled, randomized clinical trial. When the diagnosis of PE is equivocal, pulmonary angiography is the definitive study. However, it is invasive, carries a dye load, requires expertise, and is expensive.

Management

The use of anticoagulants is discussed in Chapter 3, *Heparin, Low Molecular Weight Heparin, Hirudin, and Warfarin.* Antithrombotic therapy specific for DVT and PE will be described. The initial management of a patient presenting with DVT or PE will be presented, the feasibility of outpatient management explored, and the indications for thrombolytic agents examined.

■ Deep Vein Thrombosis

Once the diagnosis of DVT has been established, the patient should be assessed as to whether the thrombosis is idiopathic or secondary to a defined risk factor such as sur-

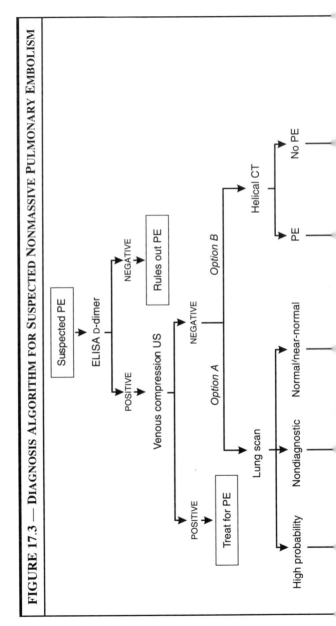

FIGURE 17.3 — DIAGNOSIS ALGORITHM FOR SUSPECTED NONMASSIVE PULMONARY EMBOLISM

Suspected PE

ELISA D-dimer

NEGATIVE → Rules out PE

POSITIVE → Venous compression US

POSITIVE → Treat for PE

NEGATIVE

Option A → Lung scan

Option B → Helical CT

High probability

Nondiagnostic

Normal/near-normal

PE

No PE

286

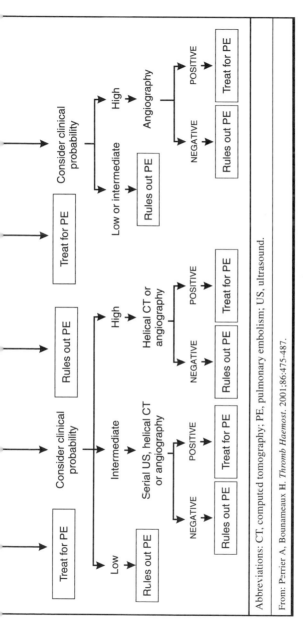

Abbreviations: CT, computed tomography; PE, pulmonary embolism; US, ultrasound.

From: Perrier A, Bounameaux H. *Thromb Haemost.* 2001;86:475-487.

17

287

gery, trauma, cancer, antiphospholipid antibody syndrome, or inherited thrombophilia. If the latter are suspected, blood samples should be obtained for measurements of proteins C and S, antithrombin, lupus anticoagulant, anticardiolipin antibody, homocysteine, and genetic testing for factor V Leiden (FVL) and the prothrombin 20210A mutation. Abnormalities noted in these tests may affect the duration of the anticoagulant treatment, but it should be noted that proteins C and S may be low during the acute phase of an illness but subsequently will return to normal. Low values of these proteins should always be confirmed by repeat testing 3 to 6 months later.

Treatment for acute DVT is usually initiated with low molecular weight heparin (LMWH). In the past 10 years, more than a dozen controlled, double-blind, clinical trials have compared various LMWHs with unfractionated heparin (UFH) in the management of acute DVT. Lensing and associates[19] performed a meta-analysis of 10 studies and noted that there was a statistically significant risk reduction in symptomatic thromboembolic complications, clinically important bleeding, and mortality with the use of LMWH.

In the early 1990s, a relatively large study of venous thrombosis treatment compared tinzaparin with UFH.[20] Over 400 patients were randomized to receive either tinzaparin 175 U/kg subcutaneously once daily or UFH infused intravenously according to the Hull protocol shown in Table 9.2. To maintain blinding of the study, patients randomized to tinzaparin received an intravenous placebo, and patients treated with UFH received a subcutaneous placebo. The activated partial thromboplastin time (aPTT) was used to monitor the heparin treatment, but the results of the test and the adjustments of heparin dose were performed by third parties not involved in the clinical management of the patients. This rigorous study design permitted an unbiased assessment of treatment outcomes. Warfarin was started on day 2 and the heparin discontinued on day 6; patients were followed for 3 months. Despite the use of intravenous UFH, new thromboembolic events occurred in 6.9% of patients assigned to UFH; the figure for tinzaparin was lower (2.8%; $P = 0.07$). While major bleeding was recorded in 5% of those receiving UFH, this complication occurred in only

0.5% of those on tinzaparin ($P = 0.006$). Finally, 21 UFH-treated patients died as compared with 10 treated with tinzaparin ($P = 0.049$). Thus, by every measure, tinzaparin was superior to UFH.

Low molecular weight heparins available in the United States are shown in Table 17.1. Two of these, enoxaparin and tinzaparin, are currently approved by the Food and Drug Administration (FDA) for the treatment of venous thrombosis. Tinzaparin is given in a once daily dose of 175 U/kg. Enoxaparin may be given either twice daily in a dose of 1 mg/kg, or once daily in a dose of 1.5 mg/kg.[21] Coincidentally with the dose of LMWH, warfarin may be started in a dose of 5 mg. This particular dose of warfarin is selected because studies by Harrison and colleagues[22] have shown that this dose is most likely to result in patient prothrombin times being in the therapeutic range by days 3 to 5. However, prothrombin time must be assessed frequently and the doses of warfarin adjusted accordingly. For example, if the INR is still only 1.2 or less on day 3 of warfarin dosing, the dose should be escalated by 2.5 mg daily until the INR is above 2.0, and then the dose can be adjusted downward. In the patient who is very sensitive to warfarin, the INR will be above 1.5 by day 2 of therapy, and the dose should be reduced by 2.5 mg. A great many factors affect sensitivity to warfarin; these include patient's diet, concomitant drugs, and mutations in the P450 cytochrome system that is responsible for warfarin metabolism.[23] While some of these factors can be anticipated (for example, meager food intake in the postoperative patient or concurrent antibiotic therapy), other factors affecting warfarin re-

TABLE 17.1 — LOW MOLECULAR WEIGHT HEPARINS USED FOR THE TREATMENT OF THROMBOEMBOLISM	
Drug (Trade)	**Dose**
Dalteparin (Fragmin)	100 U/kg q 12 h; 200 U/kg daily
Enoxaparin (Lovenox)	1 mg/kg q 12 h; 1.5 mg/kg daily
Tinzaparin (Innohep)	175 U/kg daily

17

sponsiveness may only become apparent during administration of the drug.

Low molecular weight heparin should be continued until the INR has been above 2.0 for 48 hours. This ensures that the levels of coagulation factors (prothrombin, factors VII, IX and X) have declined to sufficiently low levels that recurrent thrombosis is considered unlikely. In the majority of patients, a maintenance dose of 5 mg warfarin is satisfactory, but in young patients higher doses are usually necessary, and in elderly patients or those on restricted diets, lower doses suffice. Prothrombin times are usually obtained twice weekly until the INR consistently is in the 2 to 3 range and then biweekly or even monthly in stable patients. In those patients whose prothrombin times are quite labile, home testing of the INR may be recommended. A drop of blood, obtained from a fingerstick puncture, is presented to a machine that displays the prothrombin time and INR. This permits the patient to self-monitor the INR and in consultation with medical personnel determine the best dosing regimen compatible with the patient's lifestyle. In one study, patients performing self-testing had more INRs within the therapeutic range than patients who were on standard management.[24]

■ Outpatient Therapy

Patients with acute DVT may be treated at home if several criteria are met:

- The thrombus should be distal to the iliac vein. Iliac vein thrombi usually cause considerable leg swelling and discomfort, and frequently embolize to the lungs. Patients with such thrombi need to be managed under physician supervision until leg swelling has decreased and fear of embolization has abated; a 2 to 3 day period is appropriate.
- The presence of pulmonary emboli warrants close supervision for at least 72 hours, until the patient is hemodynamically stable and further risk of embolization has subsided.
- Patients with risk factors for bleeding, such as liver disease, peptic ulcer, and thrombocytopenia, should be given anticoagulants with great caution and in the hospital setting.

- The patient or caregiver must be instructed on the technique for administering the LMWH, and must be considered reliable.
- There must be provision for obtaining prothrombin times in the outpatient setting, since warfarin is being given concurrently with LMWH.
- The patient should be geographically accessible in the event of thrombus recurrence or an untoward reaction to the medication.
- Third-party payers must be educated about the cost-benefits of home therapy and willing to provide financial coverage for treatment.

■ Duration of Treatment

Following the transition from LMWH to warfarin, a decision must be made about the duration of oral anticoagulation. The British Thoracic Society[25] performed a study comparing 4 weeks of anticoagulation with 3 months of therapy. Approximately 350 patients were randomized to each treatment. Of those treated for 4 weeks, 7.8% had recurrent thrombosis vs 4% of those receiving anticoagulants for 3 months ($P = 0.04$), prompting a recommendation that at least 3 months of treatment be given. Prandoni et al[26] noted that the recurrence rate of DVT in patients treated for 3 months was 10% at 1 year and 20% at 2 years, suggesting that a longer treatment period might be beneficial. Six weeks of anticoagulation were compared with 6 months by Schulman et al;[27] the 6-month group had about half the recurrence rate as the 6-week group. Kearon et al[28] randomized patients to receive either 3 months or at least 6 months of anticoagulation. The study was stopped when it was observed that 17 of 83 patients whose anticoagulation was discontinued after 3 months had recurrent thromboembolism as compared with only one of 79 patients continued on anticoagulation ($P < 0.001$). Finally, a second study by Schulman et al[29] compared 6 months with treatment that was continued indefinitely in patients with a second episode of venous thromboembolism and showed a cumulative probability of recurrence of 24% vs 4% at 4 years. However, when anticoagulation is discontinued, recurrence rates are high; in the study by Agnelli and colleagues, the rate of

17

recurrence was 5% per patient-year in patients discontinuing anticoagulants after 1 year of treatment.[30]

Does this mean that anticoagulation should be continued indefinitely in all patients with DVT? The risk of bleeding must also be considered. In the Kearon study, only one patient randomized to 3 months of anticoagulation had any bleeding, as compared with nine patients in the > 6-month group ($P = 0.03$). Patients receiving anticoagulation for an indefinite period in the second Schulman study had an 8.6% risk of major hemorrhage, as compared with 2.7% in the 6-month group. Thus, bleeding becomes an important factor when anticoagulation is continued beyond 6 months.

Can the risk of recurrent thromboembolism be estimated more precisely and the duration of treatment modified accordingly? The British Thoracic Society study referred to earlier found that the subset of patients who developed thrombosis in association with a defined risk factor, such as surgery or trauma, did not have an increased rate of recurrence when treatment was stopped at 4 weeks. This important observation needs to be confirmed by a prospective randomized trial of treatment duration in persons with this particular risk factor. Are persons with inherited thrombophilia at greater risk for recurrence? In a study of patients with the prothrombin 20210A mutation, Eichinger and colleagues[31] found no increase in recurrence rates as compared with those without the mutation. Whether heterozygosity for factor V Leiden (FVL) increases recurrence rates is controversial. After 3 to 6 months of anticoagulation, Simioni and associates[32] noted that the recurrence rate in those with FVL was almost 40% at 8 years, as compared with 18% in those without the mutation. However, Eichinger et al[33] found a recurrence rate at 2 years of only 8.9% in those with FVL and 9.7% in those without, and Rintelen et al,[34] in a retrospective review, could detect no increase in rate, which was 4.8% per year for those with FVL and 5% per year in controls. Patients with hyperhomocysteinemia appear to have a high recurrence rate when anticoagulation is stopped after 6 months.[35] Whether this high recurrence rate can be lowered by decreasing serum homocysteine with folic acid treatment needs to be examined.

The following guidelines for the duration of anticoagulant therapy have been proposed by the Consensus Conference of the American College of Chest Physicians:[36]

- First event with reversible or time-limited risk factors: 3 months
- First event with idiopathic thromboembolism: 6+ months
- For patients with recurrent idiopathic thromboembolism or a continuing risk factor such as cancer, antiphospholipid antibody syndrome, or deficiency of antithrombin: 12+ months
- The duration of therapy needs to be individualized in patients with deficiency of proteins C or S, multiple thrombophilic conditions, homocysteinemia, and homozygous factor V Leiden.
- Isolated symptomatic calf vein thrombosis should be treated for at least 6 to 12 weeks. If anticoagulants are not given, serial noninvasive studies should be performed for 10 to 14 days to assess for proximal extension of the thrombus.

Complications of Deep Vein Thrombosis and Management of Pulmonary Embolism

■ Postphlebitic Syndrome

Failure of recanalization of thrombosed veins leads to the postphlebitic syndrome, which is characterized by pain and swelling of the leg and induration, discoloration, and eventually ulceration of the skin of the involved extremity. Prandoni et al[26] recorded a cumulative incidence of the postthrombotic syndrome of 22.8% after 2 years, 28% after 5 years, and 29.1% after 8 years. Franzeck et al[37] also observed post-thrombotic changes in 28% of patients in their series. The most common cause of these changes was found to be a combination of reflux and vein obstruction. This results in venous hypertension and increased flow through the superficial venous system. Chronic congestion of the skin is accompanied by thickening, pruritus, pigmentation, and ulceration.

There are several possible reasons for the development of the postphlebitic syndrome. First, thrombi located proximally in the common femoral vein or ileofemoral vein may completely obstruct venous outflow. If these thrombi do not undergo early recanalization, postphlebitic syndrome is a likely outcome. Second, recurrent episodes of DVT may eventually occlude the majority of venous outflow vessels. Finally, inadequate anticoagulation therapy during the acute episode may allow thrombus to extend to the collateral veins, further impairing venous outflow and resulting in a greater frequency of recurrent DVT.[38]

Prevention of postphlebitic syndrome requires early, intensive anticoagulation, which is continued long enough to prevent recurrent DVT (see *Duration of Treatment*, this chapter). Also, the use of compression stockings is beneficial. In a randomized trial, Brandjes and associates observed that wearing a sized-to-fit compression hose decreased the occurrence of all postphlebitic syndrome from 47% to 20%, and the severe syndrome from 23% to 11% (both *P* <0.001).[39] The stocking was worn on the involved leg beginning 2 to 3 weeks after the acute DVT and was worn during the daylight hours for up to 2 years. This is a safe and inexpensive measure that should be offered to all patients. In addition, there may be a role for fibrinolytic therapy to recanalize ileofemoral or common femoral thrombi. Three agents are currently available: streptokinase (SK), urokinase (UK), and tissue plasminogen activator (tPA).

The systemic administration of streptokinase or urokinase results in the lysis of thrombi in less than half of all patients;[40] this is because venous thrombi may be quite long and prolonged exposure to the lytic agent is required. Furthermore, major bleeding occurs in 8% to 38% with SK, much higher than the 10% with heparin therapy. With prolonged infusion of tPA (35 hrs), 40% clot lysis was achieved in four of seven patients, but 22% of all patients treated had major bleeding.[41] Even if the majority of the thrombus undergoes lysis, there may be no benefit unless the patency of the vessel is fully restored. Therefore, there have been attempts to combine lytic therapy with physical destruction of the thrombus, using catheter-directed thrombolysis. The catheter is introduced into the popliteal vein and advanced into the thrombus; the lytic agent is then sprayed into the clot. The catheter is gradually advanced and the clot lysed until flow is restored. Stents may be placed to maintain vessel patency. In a series of 312 infusions, complete lysis was achieved in 31%, and major bleeding in 11%. Pulmonary emboli occurred in 1% and there were two deaths.[42] The vein was still patent in 60% of patients at the 1-year follow-up visit. This approach is appropriate for patients with iliac or ileofemoral vein thrombosis who live near centers with the expertise to perform this sophisticated treatment. Contraindications to fibrinolytic therapy include a history of stroke, major surgery, or head injury within the past 2 weeks or any potential bleeding lesions in noncompressible areas: ie, gastrointestinal or genitourinary tract. Arterial blood gas determinations and intramuscular injections are avoided in patients receiving fibrinolytic agents.

■ **Pulmonary Embolism**

Patients with moderate PE are treated with UFH or LMWH, but those with submassive or massive PE may require fibrinolytic therapy. The decision to give a fibrinolytic agent is based on the presence of the following: hemodynamic instability with hypotension, symptomatic hypoxemia, and elevated right-heart pressure with signs of right-heart overload. When clinical suspicion of massive PE is high, one should not wait for diagnostic laboratory tests but rather immediately institute thrombolysis. In patients who are more stable, obtaining a spiral computerized tomography examination, a ventilation/perfusion scan, or a pulmonary angiogram is warranted to unequivocally establish the diagnosis of PE. An echocardiogram will confirm the presence of right-heart strain.

FDA-approved regimens for the treatment of PE are shown in Table 17.2.[43] Tissue plasminogen activator may be administered in a bolus dose of 15 mg (especially if the patient is in shock), and then 50 mg is infused over the first hour and 35 mg over the second hour for a total dose of 100 mg over 2 hours. Heparin is not given concomitantly with any fibrinolytic agent but rather is started as a continuous infusion of 500 U/hr immediately at the conclusion of fibrinolytic therapy. An aPTT is obtained and the dose of heparin adjusted to prolong the aPTT to 1.5 to 2.5 times the control value. Alternatively, LMWH may be given in full therapeutic subcutaneous doses at the conclusion of the thrombolytic treatment.

17

TABLE 17.2 — REGIMENS APPROVED BY THE FOOD AND DRUG ADMINISTRATION FOR THE TREATMENT OF PULMONARY EMBOLISM

Drug	Dose
Streptokinase	250,000 U as a loading dose over 30 min, followed by 100,000 U/hr for 24 hrs
Urokinase	4,400 U/kg as a loading dose over 10 min, followed by 4,400 U/kg/hr for 12 to 24 hrs
tPA	100 mg as a continuous intravenous infusion over 2 hrs

Abbreviation: tPA, tissue plasminogen activator.

Goldhaber SZ. In: *Disorders of Thrombosis*. Philadelphia, Pa: WB Saunders Company; 1996:321-328.

The contraindications to fibrinolytic therapy are as noted, but are all relative, depending on the severity of the PE. For example, the occurrence of a large PE in a patient with a history of stroke would not contraindicate the use of a fibrinolytic agent, as the drug may be lifesaving in this circumstance. However, it must be recognized that the risk of intracranial hemorrhage with tPA approaches 1%, which must be taken into consideration when recommending thrombolysis. It is always advisable to discuss the risks and benefits of therapy with the patient prior to embarking on a potentially dangerous course of management.

■ **Vena Caval Filters**

Insertion of a vena caval filter is an option for the prevention of venous thromboembolism. The usual indication for filter placement is the presence of a fresh thrombus in the veins of the lower extremity or pelvis in a patient unable to receive treatment doses of anticoagulants. Such patients generally have experienced major bleeding or have a strong contraindication for systemic anticoagulation. Another indication is impaired pulmonary reserve such that even a small PE could be fatal. Other, more controversial indications, are recurrent PEs despite "adequate" anticoagulation, and contraindications for other methods of prophylaxis in a patient at high risk for thromboembolism. Filters are moderately effective; the frequency of PE in patients with filters is 2.6% to 3.8%.[44] However, the frequency of DVT is 6% to 32%, and inferior vena caval thrombosis, 3.6% to 11.2%. In the only published randomized trial of filters, 400 high-risk patients received conventional anticoagulant therapy, and half the group was randomized to also have a filter placed.[45] Although the filter group had fewer PEs, at a 2-year follow-up, the frequency of DVT was almost twice as high in the filter group as in those without filters (20.8% vs 11.6%), and there was no difference in survival.

REFERENCES

1. Silverstein MD, Heit JA, Mohr DN, Petterson TM, O'Fallon WM, Melton LJ 3rd. Trends in the incidence of deep vein thrombosis and pulmonary embolism: a 25-year population-based study. *Arch Intern Med.* 1998;158:585-593.

2. Rohrer MJ. The systemic venous system: basic considerations. In: Fahey VA, ed. *Vascular Nursing.* 3rd ed. Philadelphia, Pa: WB Saunders Company; 1999:23.

3. Virchow RLK. *Thrombosis and Emboli.* Matzdorff AC, Bell WR, trans. Canton, Oh: Science History Publications; 1998:234.

4. Ryan DH, Crowther MA, Ginsberg JS, Francis CW. Relation of factor V Leiden genotype to risk for acute deep venous thrombosis after joint replacement surgery. *Ann Intern Med.* 1998;128:270-276.

5. Stewart GJ. Neutrophils and deep vein thrombosis. *Haemostasis.* 1993;23(suppl 1):127-140.

6. Wessler S, Freiman DG, Ballon JD, Katz IH, Wolff R, Wolf E. Experimental pulmonary embolism with serum-induced thrombi. *Am J Path.* 1961;38:89-101.

7. Aschwanden M, Labs KH, Engel H, et al. Acute deep vein thrombosis: early mobilization does not increase the frequency of pulmonary embolism. *Thromb Haemost.* 2001;85:42-46.

8. Anand SS, Wells PS, Hunt D, Brill-Edwards P, Cook D, Ginsberg JS. Does the patient have deep vein thrombosis [published correction appears in *JAMA.* 1998;279:1614 and 1998;280:328]? *JAMA.* 1998; 279:1094-1099.

9. Perrier A, Bounameaux H. Cost-effective diagnosis of deep vein thrombosis and pulmonary embolism. *Thromb Haemost.* 2001;86: 475-487.

10. Kearon C, Ginsberg JS, Douketis J, et al. Management of suspected deep venous thrombosis in outpatients by using clinical assessment and d-dimer testing. *Ann Intern Med.* 2001;135:108-111.

11. Perrier A, Howarth N, Didier D, et al. Performance of helical computed tomography in unselected outpatients with suspected pulmonary embolism. *Ann Intern Med.* 2001;135:88-97.

12. Wells PS, Ginsberg JS, Anderson DR, et al. Use of a clinical model for safe management of patients with suspected pulmonary embolism. *Ann Intern Med.* 1998;129:997-1005.

13. Wells PS, Anderson DR, Rodger M, et al. Excluding pulmonary embolism at the bedside without diagnostic imaging: management of patients with suspected pulmonary embolism presenting to the emergency department by using a simple clinical model and d-dimer. *Ann Intern Med.* 2001;135:98-107.

14. Kearon C, Ginsberg JS, Hirsh J. The role of venous ultrasonography in the diagnosis of suspected deep venous thrombosis and pulmonary embolism. *Ann Intern Med.* 1998;129:1044-1049.

15. Lensing AWA, Buller HR. Objective tests for the diagnosis of venous thrombosis. In: Hull R, Pineo GF, eds. *Disorders of Thrombosis.* Philadelphia, Pa: WB Saunders Company; 1995:239-257.

16. The Pioped Investigators. Value of the ventilation/perfusion scan in acute pulmonary embolism. Results of the prospective investigation of pulmonary embolism diagnosis (PIOPED). *JAMA.* 1990;263: 2753-2759.

17. Rathbun SW, Raskob GE, Whitsett TL. Sensitivity and specificity of helical computed tomography in the diagnosis of pulmonary embolism: a systematic review. *Ann Intern Med.* 2000;132:227-232.

18. Mullins MD, Becker DM, Hagspiel KD, Philbrick JT. The role of spiral volumetric computed tomography in the diagnosis of pulmonary embolism. *Arch Intern Med.* 2000;160:293-298.

19. Lensing AW, Prins MH, Davidson BL, Hirsh J. Treatment of deep venous thrombosis with low-molecular-weight heparins. A meta-analysis. *Arch Intern Med.* 1995;155:601-607.

20. Hull RD, Raskob GE, Pineo GF, et al. Subcutaneous low-molecular-weight heparin compared with continuous intravenous heparin in the treatment of proximal-vein thrombosis. *N Engl J Med.* 1992;326:975-982.

21. Merli G, Spiro TE, Olsson CG, et al. Subcutaneous enoxaparin once or twice daily compared with intravenous unfractionated heparin for treatment of venous thromboembolic disease. *Ann Intern Med*. 2001;134:191-202.

22. Harrison L, Johnston M, Massicotte MP, Crowther M, Moffat K, Hirsh J. Comparison of 5-mg and 10-mg loading doses in initiation of warfarin therapy. *Ann Intern Med*. 1997;126:133-136.

23. Aithal GP, Day CP, Kesteven PKL, Daly AK. Association of polymorphisms in the cytochrome P450 CYP2C9 with warfarin dose requirement and risk of bleeding complications. *Lancet*. 1999;353:717-719.

24. Watzke HH, Forberg E, Svolba G, Jimenez-Boj E, Krinninger B. A prospective controlled trial comparing weekly self-testing and self-dosing with the standard management of patients on stable oral anticoagulation. *Thromb Haemost*. 2000;83:661-665.

25. Research Committee of the British Thoracic Society. Optimum duration of anticoagulation for deep-vein thrombosis and pulmonary embolism. *Lancet*. 1992;340:873-876.

26. Prandoni P, Lensing AW, Cogo A, et al. The long-term clinical course of acute deep venous thrombosis. *Ann Intern Med*. 1996;125:1-7.

27. Schulman S, Rhedin AS, Lindmarker P, et al. A comparison of six weeks with six months of oral anticoagulant therapy after a first episode of venous thromboembolism. Duration of Anticoagulation Trial Study Group. *N Engl J Med*. 1995;332:1661-1665.

28. Kearon C, Gent M, Hirsh J, et al. A comparison of three months of anticoagulation with extended anticoagulation for a first episode of idiopathic venous thromboembolism [published correction appears in *N Engl J Med*. 1999;341:298]. *N Engl J Med*. 1999;340:901-907.

29. Schulman S, Granqvist S, Holmstrom M, et al. The duration of oral anticoagulant therapy after a second episode of venous thromboembolism. Duration of Anticoagulation Trial Study Group. *N Engl J Med*. 1997;336:393-398.

30. Agnelli G, Prandoni P, Santamaria MB, et al. Three months versus one year of oral anticoagulant therapy for idiopathic deep venous thrombosis. *N Engl J Med*. 2001;345:165-169.

31. Eichinger S, Minar E, Hirschl M, et al. The risk of early recurrent venous thromboembolism after oral anticoagulant therapy in patients with the G20210A transition in the prothrombin gene. *Thromb Haemost*. 1999;81:14-17.

32. Simioni P, Prandoni P, Lensing AW, et al. The risk of recurrent venous thromboembolism in patients with an Arg[506] to Gln mutation in the gene for factor V (factor V Leiden). *N Engl J Med*. 1997;336:399-403.

33. Eichinger S, Pabinger I, Stumpflen A, et al. The risk of recurrent venous thromboembolism in patients with and without factor V Leiden. *Thromb Haemost.* 1997;77:624-628.

34. Rintelen C, Pabinger I, Knobl P, Lechner K, Mannhalter C. Probability of recurrence of thrombosis in patients with and without factor V Leiden. *Thromb Haemost.* 1996;75:229-232.

35. Eichinger S, Stumpflen A, Hirschl M, et al. Hyperhomocysteinemia is a risk factor of recurrent venous thromboembolism. *Thromb Haemost.* 1998;80:566-569.

36. Hyers TM, Agnelli G, Hull RD, et al. Antithrombotic therapy for venous thromboembolic disease. *Chest.* 2001;119(suppl):176S-209S.

37. Franzeck UK, Schalch I, Bollinger A. On the relationship between changes in the deep veins evaluated by duplex sonography and the postthrombotic syndrome 12 years after deep vein thrombosis. *Thromb Haemost.* 1997;77:1109-1112.

38. Hull RD, Raskob GE, Brant RF, Pineo GF, Valentine KA. Relation between the time to achieve the lower limit of the APTT therapeutic range and recurrent venous thromboembolism during heparin treatment for deep vein thrombosis. *Arch Intern Med.* 1997;157:2562-2568.

39. Brandjes DPM, Buller HR, Heijboer H, et al. Randomised trial of effect of compression stockings in patients with symptomatic proximal-vein thrombosis. *Lancet.* 1997;349:759-762.

40. Kwaan HC. Thrombolytic therapy for deep vein thrombosis. *J Lab Clin Med.* 1992;119:450-451. Editorial.

41. Marder VJ, Brenner B, Totterman S, et al. Comparison of dosage schedules of rt-PA in the treatment of proximal deep vein thrombosis. *J Lab Clin Med.* 1992;119:485-495.

42. Mewissen MW, Seabrook GR, Meissner MH, Cynamon J, Labropoulos N, Haughton SH. Catheter-directed thrombolysis for lower extremity deep venous thrombosis: report of a national multicenter registry. *Radiology.* 1999;211:39-49.

43. Goldhaber SZ. Thrombolytic therapy for venous thromboembolism. In: Hull R, Pineo GF, eds. *Disorders of Thrombosis.* Philadelphia, Pa: WB Saunders Company; 1995:321-328.

44. Streiff MB. Vena caval filters: a comprehensive review. *Blood.* 2000;95:3669-3677.

45. Decousus H, Leizorovicz A, Parent F, et al. A clinical trial of vena caval filters in the prevention of pulmonary embolism in patients with proximal deep-vein thrombosis. *N Engl J Med.* 1998;338:409-415.

18 Complications of Antithrombotic Therapy

Introduction

The major complication of antithrombotic therapy is bleeding. Most of the agents in current clinical use have a narrow therapeutic index, ie, the ratio of the toxic dose to the effective dose for a therapeutic effect is small. Therefore, patients receiving these agents must be closely supervised and many of the drugs require laboratory monitoring. Because of these considerations, there has been a great impetus to develop safer agents that do not need laboratory control. Many of these drugs are currently in clinical trials. Table 18.1 lists the adverse reactions associated with antithrombotic agents.

Warfarin

Hemorrhage is the most common adverse effect associated with warfarin administration. To predict the risk of bleeding, Beyth and colleagues[1] developed a five-point scoring system, with one point given for each of the following:

- Age >65
- History of stroke
- History of gastrointestinal bleeding
- Specific comorbid conditions (recent myocardial infarction [MI], elevated serum creatinine, hematocrit <30%, or diabetes)

Low-risk patients had a score of 0; intermediate-risk patients, 1 or 2; and high-risk, 3 or 4. The risk of bleeding in these three groupings at 12 months was 3%, 8%, and 30%. A Mayo Clinic study observed that malignancy was also a risk factor for bleeding, but that age, sex, history of gastrointestinal hemorrhage, peptic ulcer, alcohol abuse, hypertension, and stroke were not associated with major bleeding.[2] This discrepancy in study outcomes reflects the fact

18

TABLE 18.1 — ADVERSE REACTIONS ASSOCIATED WITH ANTITHROMBOTIC AGENTS

Adverse Effect	Warfarin	Heparin	LMWH	Fibrinolytics	Antiplatelet
Bleeding	Yes	Yes	Yes	Yes	Yes
Thrombocytopenia	No	1% to 3%	< 1%	No	Abciximab-1%; Ticlopidine-1%
Skin/muscle necrosis	Yes	Yes	Rare	No	No
Osteoporosis	?No	Yes	Rare	No	No
Alopecia	Yes	Yes	Rare	No	No
Other	No	Eosinophilia; hypoaldosteronism; elevated transaminases	No	No	No

Abbreviation: LMWH, low molecular weight heparin.

that the risk of bleeding with warfarin treatment is multi-factorial (Table 18.2). In addition, and perhaps most important, outcomes are related to the experience and expertise of those giving this anticoagulant. Several studies have noted that complications are far less frequent in patients managed by coordinated anticoagulation clinics.[3]

TABLE 18.2 — FACTORS INFLUENCING THE RISK OF WARFARIN-INDUCED BLEEDING

- Age
- Diet
- Medications
- Changes in therapy
- Duration of therapy
- Concurrent diseases
- Genetic polymorphisms

■ **Genetic Factors**

Warfarin (S-component) is metabolized by the P450 cytochrome (CYP) 2C9 of the liver. There are two allelic variants of CYP 2C9, and these are much less efficient in metabolizing warfarin than the wild-type cytochrome. Patients with these alleles require lower doses of warfarin to achieve an anticoagulant effect and because of their increased sensitivity to the drug, are more likely to experience bleeding complications.[4] Since most patients requiring warfarin are unlikely to be tested for the presence of these cytochrome alleles, it would seem prudent to initiate warfarin therapy with a relatively low dose of 5 mg. Harrison and colleagues showed that when 10 mg was used as the starting dose, patients were significantly more likely to be over-anticoagulated than when they were given 5 mg.[5] At 60 hours after the initiation of warfarin therapy, nine of 25 patients in the 10-mg group, but none of the 24 patients in the 5-mg group, had international normalized ratios (INRs) over 3.0. Four of the patients in the 10-mg group eventually required vitamin K because of excessive anticoagulation.

18

■ Diet

The antagonist of warfarin, vitamin K, is found in fresh vegetables, butter, oils, meat products, and avocado.[6] Therefore, the composition of the diet will have an important influence on the intensity of treatment. In one study of patients who had been poorly controlled on oral anticoagulants, administration of a diet of known vitamin K composition resulted in more stable anticoagulation.[7] Diet is especially important in patients with concurrent illnesses, whose nutrition may be marginal. These patients have heightened sensitivity to warfarin and an increased risk of anticoagulant-associated bleeding. On the other hand, the use of enteral supplements containing vitamin K promotes resistance to warfarin. Prior to initiating warfarin therapy, the nutritional status of the patient should be assessed and the doses of warfarin correspondingly adjusted.

■ Drugs

Many commonly used medications have significant interactions with warfarin. In 1994, Wells and associates[8] (Table 3.5) reviewed all reports of warfarin-drug interactions and found original reports of 186 such interactions. Potentiation of warfarin effect was observed with six antibiotics, five cardiac drugs, two anti-inflammatory agents, two histamine$_2$-blockers, and alcohol in persons with concomitant liver disease (Table 18.3). Inhibition of warfarin effect was noted with three antibiotics, three central nervous system (CNS) drugs, cholestyramine, and sucralfate. Since that time, an important interaction between acetaminophen and warfarin was recognized,[9] and it has also been suggested that certain herbal remedies, such as ginkgo biloba, ginseng, and garlic, may enhance the effects of warfarin. In general, patients should be alerted to the possibility of warfarin-drug interactions. They should notify their caregivers whenever there is a change in their diet or medications. INR measurements should be performed during the period of potential drug interaction and the dosage of warfarin adjusted to assure that prothrombin times remain within the therapeutic range.

TABLE 18.3 — DRUG-WARFARIN INTERACTIONS

Drug	Potentiate	Inhibit
Antibiotics	Cotrimoxazole Erythromycin Fluconazole Isoniazid Metronidazole Miconazole Ciprofloxacin	Griseofulvin Rifampin Nafcillin
Cardiac drugs	Clofibrate Propafenone Propranolol Sulfinpyrazone	—
Antipyretics, Anti-inflammatories	Acetaminophen Phenybutazone Piroxicam	—
Histamine$_2$-blockers	Cimetidine Omeprazole	—
Central nervous system agents	—	Barbiturates Carbamazepine Chlordiazepoxide
Other	Lovastatin Simvastatin	Cholestyramine Androgens Sucralfate

- **Changes and Duration of Warfarin Treatment**

A study of 96 patients followed for up to 23 years showed that thromboembolism occurred most often during periods of high variability in the prothrombin time ratios.[10] A decline in the INR to less than 1.5 increases the frequency of thrombotic events to as high as 17.5%, as compared with 2.3% for INRs within the 2 to 3 range.[11] Instability of the prothrombin time may occur because of changes in diet or medications, poor compliance, or interruption of anticoagulation for any reason. The latter is usually engendered by the need for an invasive procedure. However, it should be recognized that certain types of surgery, such as cataract extraction and dental procedures, do not require cessation of anticoagulation. The main risk in these operations is related to the method of administration of the anesthetic agent; retrobulbar injections or lingual nerve blocks may be associated with hematoma formation. If such injections are required or if more extensive procedures are undertaken, warfarin should be withheld for approximately 4 days to allow the INR to decline to below 1.5;[12,13] this level does not increase bleeding. The warfarin may be resumed on the evening of surgery. Heparin needs to be given preoperatively only if venous or arterial thrombosis has occurred within the past month, and it need not be started until the INR is below 2. Postoperatively, patients will need anticoagulant prophylaxis, given either intravenously or subcutaneously, depending on thrombosis risk, and continued until an INR of 2 or more is sustained for at least 48 hours.

Several recent studies have emphasized that warfarin therapy for conditions such as atrial fibrillation and recurrent venous thromboembolism should be continued for many months, if not indefinitely. This long duration of oral anticoagulation increases the risk for bleeding. Using the prediction rule described previously, Beyth and colleagues[14] observed that patients prospectively classified into low-, medium-, and high-risk categories had cumulative incidences of bleeding at 48 months of 3%, 12%, and 53%, respectively.

■ Management of Warfarin-Induced Bleeding

The first step in the management of bleeding in patients taking warfarin is to stop the drug. However, recovery of clotting factor levels may take several days, depending upon the vitamin K content of the patient's diet. To rapidly raise coagulant factor concentrations in patients with life-threatening hemorrhage, clotting factor concentrates are given.[15] The older concentrates were plasma-derived and consisted mainly of prothrombin complex factors. They had the disadvantages of thrombogenicity and potential for transmission of infectious agents. More recently, recombinant factor VIIa (NovoSeven) has been used with excellent control of bleeding, although thrombosis risk remains a concern. Fresh frozen plasma is an alternative therapy but usually does not completely correct the prothrombin time.

Doses of at least 20 mL/kg are needed to raise clotting factor levels above 20% of normal; such doses carry a substantial risk of producing circulatory overload. After an initial bolus of 200 mL, plasma may be given as a continuous infusion of 100 mL/hr with monitoring of venous pressure and administration of diuretics. Recently, plasma treated to inactivate infectious agents has become available.

Patients with warfarin-induced bleeding should also receive vitamin K, but the doses should be adjusted according to the intensity of bleeding. If bleeding is major, 5 mg to 10 mg of vitamin K is given subcutaneously. However, in most patients who do not have serious bleeding episodes and have an INR of less than 10, an oral dose of 2.5 mg vitamin K decreases the INR to between 2 and 4 by 48 hours.[16] And in nonbleeding patients, doses as low as 1 mg given by mouth reliably reduce the INR to the therapeutic range within 24 hours.[17]

■ Adverse Reactions Other Than Bleeding

Skin and muscle necrosis is a dreaded complication of warfarin therapy. The pathogenesis is related to the effect of warfarin on the levels of proteins C and S. Because these anticoagulant proteins disappear at a faster rate than prothrombin, an imbalance between procoagulant and anticoagulant proteins transiently develops. A recent investigation showed that prothrombin protects activated factor V (aFV) from degradation by activated protein C.[18] Low levels of protein C in the face of normal prothrombin concentrations is predictive of less inactivation of aFV with resultant hypercoagulability. The clinical manifestations of this disorder are necrosis of skin and fat, especially in such areas as the breast and abdominal wall. In addition, the veins of the lower extremities may become thrombosed, leading to venous gangrene.

This devastating syndrome is prevented by avoiding the use of warfarin in patients with low baseline levels of proteins C and S; such patients are those with inherited deficiencies of these factors (detected by a positive personal or family history of thrombosis), patients suffering from poor nutrition (including those who are unable to eat because of gastrointestinal disease, recent surgery, or neurologic disease), and patients with heparin-induced thromb-

18

ocytopenia (HIT) (see below). In patients with hereditary deficiencies of proteins C or S, warfarin is introduced when therapeutic levels of heparin or low molecular weight heparin (LMWH) have been achieved. In other patients, warfarin therapy is delayed until the patient's nutrition improves, or the HIT has resolved; the starting dose should not exceed 5 mg daily. In patients who are receiving warfarin, the syndrome may be recognized by the development of skin discoloration and pain in a very localized body area and strongly suspected if the prothrombin time becomes greatly elevated with a single dose of warfarin, indicating extreme sensitivity of the vitamin–K-dependent proteins to the vitamin K antagonist. The warfarin should be stopped immediately and the patient treated with vitamin K; in severe cases it is recommended that activated protein C, if available, or fresh frozen plasma be infused as a source of proteins C and S. A parenteral anticoagulant, such as heparin, LMWH, or recombinant hirudin, should also be given.

Another unusual complication of warfarin treatment is the "purple toes" syndrome. Patients with this syndrome usually have severe aortoiliac atheromatous disease; warfarin administration appears to promote plaque destabilization with distal embolization of cholesterol crystals, especially to the toes. Cessation of warfarin therapy generally resolves the problem, but vascular surgery may be necessary if there is extensive disease.[19]

Alopecia is an infrequent occurrence in patients on warfarin therapy. In two patients, hair loss was decreased with ubidecarenone (Coenzyme Q10), 30 mg daily.[20] Another potential but as yet undocumented complication of warfarin usage is osteoporosis. Warfarin effects osteocalcin, a vitamin K–dependent protein required for maintenance of bone matrix. Reassuringly, a recent study of 149 elderly women taking warfarin found no differences in bone mineral density as compared with age–, weight–, and estrogen–use-matched control subjects.[21]

The teratogenicity of warfarin is well recognized. The greatest risk is from week 6 to week 12 of gestation, but central nervous system malformations may occur later. During the third trimester, there is a risk of intracranial bleeding in the fetus. Therefore, warfarin should be discontinued when pregnancy is recognized in women who are taking the drug and alternative anticoagulation with heparin or LMWH substituted.[22] Warfarin may be resumed in the immediate postpartum period, even in women who nurse. Although some warfarin may appear in breast milk, the amounts are small and are counteracted by the vitamin K which is routinely given newborns at birth.

Heparin and Low Molecular Weight Heparin

The use of unfractionated heparin (UFH) and LMWH is associated with a variety of complications; as with warfarin, the most frequent is bleeding. However, other serious adverse effects also occur; these include HIT, osteoporosis, and less commonly eosinophilia, alopecia, and transaminitis.

■ **Bleeding**

At the Sixth Consensus Conference on Antithrombotic Therapy, it was estimated that major bleeding occurs in from 0% to 7% of patients receiving intravenous (IV) UFH, and the rate of fatal bleeding is up to 2%.[23] For LMWH, the rates are 0% to 3.0% and up to 0.8%, respectively. Thus, LMWH appears to be associated with a lesser risk of serious hemorrhage. One reason for this relates to the greater complexity of giving UFH. While LMWH is injected subcutaneously, UFH is usually given IV, requiring solution preparation, infusion pumps, and frequent laboratory monitoring. Errors have been discovered with infusion-pump precision, in making up solutions, in infusion and charting techniques, and with interruptions of infusions,[24] as well as with variations in the sensitivity to heparin of the partial thromboplastin time reagents in current use. Other pharmacologic problems with UFH, such as dose-dependent absorption and half-life, may likewise lead to under- or over-anticoagulation. LMWH is well-absorbed at any dose and the anticoagulant effect is highly predictable.

Kitchens reviewed the sites of bleeding related to UH or LMWH therapy in 474 patients.[25] Most common is wound and soft tissue hemorrhage (31%), followed by gastrointestinal (27%) and genitourinary (19%) bleeding. Less frequent (about 2%), but of great importance, is bleeding into the central nervous system, retroperitoneum, and adrenal glands. The clinical manifestations of adrenal hemorrhage may be very subtle, with only generalized weakness, hypotension, and hyperkalemia pointing to bleeding in these organs. A major predisposing factor to bleeding appears to be the overall health of the patient, with those in good physical condition having a 2% frequency, whereas those who are severely ill having a 25% incidence.[26,27] Frail, elderly women in particular seem to be susceptible to heparin-associated hemorrhages, and such bleeding appears to occur with equal frequency with either UH or LMWH.

Another important bleeding complication is spinal subarachnoid hematoma. This subject was reviewed in 1986; 33 patients were reported to have bleeding after attempted lumbar puncture.[28] Six had received heparin alone, and another six both heparin and warfarin. With intensive anticoagulant prophylaxis for orthopedic surgery and the widespread use of epidural anesthesia, many more cases of spinal epidural hematoma are now recognized.[29] As a consequence of this experience, guidelines for the use of anesthetic and anticoagulant agents have been established[30] (Table 18.4). As noted for other types of bleeding, most epidural hematomas have been in elderly women who should be given anticoagulants with considerable caution and close monitoring.

■ **Management of Bleeding Due to Heparins**

Bleeding in patients receiving heparin is managed by discontinuing the agent. Often this is all that is necessary, because the short half-life of the drug (90 minutes) ensures that the anticoagulant effect will disappear rapidly. However, if serious bleeding begins immediately after a dose is given or the patient has delayed heparin clearance (because of renal or hepatic disease), it may be necessary to neutralize the heparin with protamine. The dose is 1 mg for each 100 U of heparin suspected to be in the circulation; in practice, giving half this dose is usually safe and effective and can be repeated if necessary. Overdosing protamine may cause hypotension and even bleeding; allergic reactions to the drug have also been reported.

Reversal of LMWH is more challenging, since LMWH has a longer half-life and is less susceptible to inactivation

TABLE 18.4 — GUIDELINES FOR THE USE OF ANESTHETICS AND ANTICOAGULANTS IN PATIENTS UNDERGOING SURGERY

- Anti-Xa levels are not predictive of bleeding risk; therefore, monitoring is not recommended
- Antiplatelet or oral anticoagulant medications given in combination with low molecular weight heparin (LMWH) increase the risk of bleeding. The patient-care team should be educated regarding the dangers of this combination
- Traumatic needle or catheter placement may increase the risk of bleeding with a LMWH
- In patients who have had preoperative LMWH, a single dose spinal anesthetic may be safest, and should be given no earlier than 10 to 12 hours after a prophylactic dose, and 24 hours after a therapeutic dose of LMWH
- In patients who are to have postoperative LMWH, indwelling catheters are removed the day after surgery, and the first dose of LMWH is given 2 hours after catheter removal
- If LMWH is given during continuous anesthesia with an indwelling catheter, an opioid or dilute local anesthetic solution is recommended and frequent monitoring of neurological function is essential. Catheter removal should be delayed for at least 10 to 12 hours after a dose of LMWH, and the subsequent dose of LMWH is given no sooner than 2 hours after catheter removal

Horlocker TT, Wedel DJ. Neuraxial block and low-molecular-weight heparin: balancing perioperative analgesia and thromboprophylaxis. *Reg Anesth Pain Med* 1998;23(suppl 2).164-177.

by protamine. In a study of the neutralizing effects of protamine on UFH and LMWH, Wolzt et al[31] found that a dose of 1 mg/100 anti-Xa U of LMWH almost completely reversed the prolongation of the activated partial thromboplastin time (aPTT) and thrombin time, but had only a weak effect on anti-Xa activity. However, since the subjects they studied were healthy volunteers, it is not known whether correction of the anti-Xa activity would be needed to control bleeding or whether normalization of the aPTT and thrombin time is sufficient.

■ Heparin-Induced Thrombocytopenia

Heparin-induced thrombocytopenia is a devastating complication that occurs in about 1% to 3% of patients who receive IVUFH, but in no more than 0.1% of patients treated with LMWH.[32] HIT is due to the formation of antibodies against a complex of heparin and platelet factor 4.[33] When these complexes attach to the membranes of platelets or endothelial cells, they provoke platelet activation, release of vasoconstrictors, formation of platelet microparticles, and exposure of tissue factor. The consequence of these effects is vascular occlusion due to platelet masses and fibrin (the white-clot syndrome). MI, ischemic stroke, peripheral artery occlusion, pulmonary embolism, and venous gangrene have all been reported. The diagnosis is based on the clinical history of prolonged or repeated exposure to heparin, a rapid decline in platelet count (which may still be in the normal range), and either a new thrombotic episode or worsening of existing thrombosis. Confirmation of the diagnosis requires laboratory testing using either a platelet-aggregation assay, the serotonin-release test, or an enzyme-linked immunoabsorbent assay.

Treatment includes immediate cessation of all forms of heparin, including LMWH; the latter invariably cross-reacts with the antibodies. Effective anticoagulation must be given, otherwise thrombosis is progressive. Warfarin is contraindicated because levels of protein C in these patients are low, increasing their susceptibility to warfarin-tissue necrosis (venous limb gangrene).[34] Several agents are available; they include lepirudin (Refludan) and argatroban, which do not cross-react with the HIT antibodies, and danaparoid (Orgaran), which has a 10% cross-reactivity with the antibodies.[35] Dosing guidelines are presented in Table 18.5. Warfarin may be initiated when the platelet count is rising and it is clear that the patient is out of danger. Doses not exceeding 5 mg daily are suggested. Since both lepirudin and argatroban inhibit thrombin, they prolong the prothrombin time as well as the thrombin time. This complicates using the INR to monitor warfarin therapy. The INR can be estimated using the mathematical expression

TABLE 18.5 — ANTICOAGULANT THERAPY IN PATIENTS WITH HEPARIN-INDUCED THROMBOCYTOPENIA

Agent	Dose and Monitoring
Lepirudin	• IV bolus of 0.4 mg/kg • Continuous infusion of 0.15 mg/kg/h • Monitor with aPTT; do baseline and repeat 4 hours after initiation: ratio to normal should be 1.5-to-2.5 • Check aPTT at least twice daily during therapy • Reduce dose by 50% or more if renal failure present
Argatroban	• Continuous IV infusion of 2 µg/kg/min • Check aPTT 4 hours after initiation and adjust dose until target aPTT of 1.5 to 3.0 times control is attained • Reduce dose by 0.5 µg/kg/min if epatic impairment
Danaparoid	• IV bolus of 2500 U • Then, 400 U/h × 4 hours; 300 U/h × 4 hours • Then, 200 U/h as continuous infusion • Monitor platelet count; if renal failure, obtain anti-Xa level during treatment (should not exceed 1 U/mL)

Abbreviations: aPTT, activated partial thromboplastin time; IV, intravenous.

available in the argatroban dosing guidelines, or one can gradually decrease the dose of the thrombin inhibitor beginning 3 days after the initiation of warfarin therapy in anticipation of progressive lengthening of the prothrombin time by warfarin.

A localized form of HIT, presenting as skin necrosis at the sites of injection of either UFH or LMWH, is also recognized and responds to cessation of heparin therapy. A vivid photograph of heparin-induced skin necrosis was published in the *New England Journal of Medicine* (1996;335:

18

715). Lastly, it should be noted that heparin-induced plate-let antibodies are transient; in the study of Warkentin and Kelton,[36] antibodies fell to undetectable levels at a median of 50 to 85 days after the initial event. Brief re-exposure to heparin after this time, in both their study and that of Potzsch and associates[37] appeared to be safe. However, such re-exposure should only be done if there is a compelling indication such as cardiac surgery and the exposure time limited to just the time of operation. Testing for heparin an-tibodies should be performed using sensitive assays both prior to and following heparin administration. Early recog-nition and prompt treatment of HIT maybe lifesaving and limb-sparing.

■ Osteoporosis

Unfractionated heparin has been found to impair bone deposition and accelerate bone resorption, whereas LMWH only impedes bone deposition.[38] Furthermore, concentra-tions of LMWH 6- to 8-fold higher than those of UFH were required to inhibit osteoblast function *in vitro*.[39] The over-all frequency of osteoporosis is somewhat less than 5% with UFH and lower with LMWH. It appears to occur more fre-quently with higher doses given for prolonged periods. Walenga and Bick[40] recommend that if the duration of therapy is greater than 12 months and the dose is 20,000 U daily or less, or if the duration is 3 months or less but the dose is greater than 20,000 U daily, then baseline bone den-sitometry should be obtained and calcium supplements con-sidered.

■ Other Reactions

Eosinophilia occurs fairly commonly (estimates range from 10% to 50% in those exposed for long periods of time) and may be associated with eczematous plaques at injec-tion sites.[41] More severe reactions, such as hypotension, chest pain, and shortness of breath, are probably manifes-tations of HIT. Alopecia occurs in less than 1% of patients. Patients will often show evidence of suppression of aldos-terone secretion, manifested by hyperkalemia. A patient tak-ing heparin subcutaneously for 4 years had hypo-aldosteronism and at autopsy had thinning of the adrenal cortex.[42] Hyperkalemia also occurs during therapy with

LMWH.[43] During heparin treatment, serum transaminase levels may double, but there is no histologic evidence of liver damage, and other tests of liver function remain within the normal range.

■ **Heparin During Pregnancy**

Unfractionated heparin and LMWH may be safely given during pregnancy; they do not cross the placenta or appear in the maternal milk. However, pregnant patients taking heparin are at risk for all of the complications listed above. Prolongation of the aPTT may persist despite cessation of heparin 12 hours prior to predicted delivery, and serious bleeding has been reported.[44] Heparin should be discontinued at least 24 to 36 hours prior to labor induction, and the aPTT checked to ascertain whether it has returned to the normal range. In patients receiving heparin because of thromboembolic events during previous pregnancies, stopping heparin for 1 to 2 days prior to delivery is unlikely to result in recurrent thrombosis. However, it is important to resume anticoagulation soon after delivery because the risk of new thrombosis is greatest during the first 6 weeks postpartum.

Pregnancy is associated with bone loss, and this is aggravated by heparin exposure. Otherwise unexplained back pain may be the earliest sign of impending vertebral fracture. Douketis and associates[45] performed a prospective, matched cohort study in pregnant women, and found that long-term heparin treatment was associated with a significant reduction in bone density which did not correlate with the dose or duration of heparin exposure. Other studies have shown that LMWH causes less bone loss than UFH. Nevertheless, all pregnant women receiving heparin should be informed about the risks of bone loss and the possibility of fractures. Whether calcium supplementation and the use of calcitonin or other agents will be safe and effective in these women needs to be investigated.

Fibrinolytic Agents

Loscalzo[46] lists three principal shortcomings of fibrinolytic therapy:
• Bleeding

18

- Delayed lysis
- Reocclusion.

Serious bleeding occurs in about 1% of patients but may be intracranial and lead to considerable disability and even death. In 71,000 patients with MI treated with tissue plasminogen activator (tPA), the frequency of intracranial bleeding was 0.95%; 53% died during hospitalization and another 25% had residual neurologic deficit.[47] The major risk factors for bleeding were older age, female gender, black ethnicity, systolic blood pressure of 140 mm Hg or more, history of stroke, tPA dose more than 1.5 mg/kg, and lower body weight. In another study of 20,768 patients receiving either tPA or streptokinase (SK), the frequency of strokes was 1.14%; 0.36% were hemorrhagic, 0.48% were ischemic, and 0.3% were not further defined.[48] Patients treated with tPA had a small but significant excess of stroke as compared with those who received SK (1.33% vs 0.94%).

Any interruption of vascular integrity in a patient receiving fibrinolytic agents may lead to hemorrhage; for example, concurrent invasive procedures, such as coronary angioplasty and pulmonary artery catheter insertion, may result in hematoma formation at access sites. Gastrointestinal and retroperitoneal hemorrhage are also reported. Bleeding is due to the fibrinolytic activity of plasmin and also to the effects of fibrin degradation products, which interfere with platelet aggregation and fibrinogen polymerization.

Delayed lysis may be due to the depletion of plasminogen, which is the zymogen for plasmin. This may be due to consumption coagulopathy or prolonged administration of lytic agents and is corrected by plasma infusions. Several studies have shown that thrombolysis induces paradoxical activation of coagulation.[49] Plasmin can activate platelets and promote factor X activation. Furthermore, thrombin bound to fibrin may be exposed in the crevices of fissured plaques, where it may stimulate continued fibrin deposition. The consequences of this thrombin exposure are reocclusion of vessels in patients who initially had successful thrombolysis. Heparin is unable to neutralize clot-bound thrombin; inactivation requires direct thrombin inhibitors such as hirudin.

Complications unique to SK include fever, allergic reactions, and hypotension. A trial of anisolated human plasminogen streptokinase activator complex (anistreplase) was discontinued because several patients had severe hypotension,[50] possibly related to dose and infusion rate. In some patients, preformed antibodies to SK may dampen the response, although the doses of SK usually employed are sufficiently high to overcome most antibodies.

REFERENCES

1. Beyth RJ, Quinn LM, Landefeld CS. Prospective evaluation of an index for predicting the risk of major bleeding in outpatients treated with warfarin. *Am J Med*. 1998;105:91-99.

2. Gitter MJ, Jaeger TM, Petterson TM, Gersh BJ, Silverstein MD. Bleeding and thromboembolism during anticoagulant therapy: a population-based study in Rochester, Minnesota. *Mayo Clin Proc*. 1995;70:725-733.

3. Poller L, Shiach CR, MacCallum PK, et al. Multicentre randomised study of computerised anticoagulant dosage. European Concerted Action on Anticoagulation. *Lancet*. 1998;352:1505-1509.

4. Aithal GP, Day CP, Kesteven PJ, Daly AK. Association of polymorphisms in the cytochrome P450 CYP2C9 with warfarin dose requirement and risk of bleeding complications. *Lancet*. 1999;353:717-719.

5. Harrison L, Johnston M, Massicotte MP, Crowther M, Moffat K, Hirsh J. Comparison of 5-mg and 10-mg loading doses in initiation of warfarin therapy. *Ann Intern Med*. 1997;126:133-136.

6. Blickstein D, Shaklai M, Inbal A. Warfarin antagonism by avocado. *Lancet*. 1991;337:914-915. Letter.

7. Marongiu F, Sorano GG, Conti M, et al. Known vitamin K intake and management of poorly controlled oral anticoagulant therapy. *Lancet*. 1992;340:545-546. Letter.

8. Wells PS, Holbrook AM, Crowther NR, Hirsh J. Interactions of warfarin with drugs and food. *Ann Intern Med*. 1994;121:676-683.

9. Hylek EM, Heiman H, Skates SJ, Sheehan MA, Singer DE. Acetaminophen and other risk factors for excessive warfarin anticoagulation. *JAMA*. 1998;279:657-662.

10. Huber KC, Gersh BJ, Bailey KR, et al. Variability in anticoagulation control predicts thromboembolism after mechanical cardiac valve replacement. a 23-year population-based study. *Mayo Clin Proc*. 1997;72:1103-1110.

18

11. Palareti G, Manotti C, D'Angelo A, et al. Thrombotic events during oral anticoagulant treatment: results of the inception-cohort, prospective, collaborative ISCOAT study: ISCOAT Study Group (Italian Study on complications of Oral Anticoagulant Therapy). *Thromb Haemost*. 1997;78:1438-1443.

12. White RH, McKittrick T, Hutchinson R, Twitchell J. Temporary discontinuation of warfarin therapy: changes in the international normalized ratio. *Ann Intern Med*. 1995;122:40-42.

13. Kearon C, Hirsh J. Management of anticoagulation before and after elective surgery. *N Engl J Med*. 1997;336:1506-1511.

14. Beyth RJ, Quinn LM, Landefeld CS. Prospective evaluation of an index for predicting risk of major bleeding in outpatients treated with warfarin. *Am J Med*. 1998;105:91-99.

15. Makris M, Greaves M, Phillips WS, Kitchen S, Rosendaal FR, Preston FE. Emergency oral anticoagulant reversal: the relative efficacy of infusions of fresh frozen plasma and clotting factor concentrate on correction of the coagulopathy. *Thromb Haemost*. 1997;77: 477-480.

16. Weibert RT, Le DT, Kayser SR, Rapaport SI. Correction of excessive anticoagulation with low-dose oral vitamin K_1. *Ann Intern Med*. 1997;125:959-962.

17. Crowther MA, Donovan D, Harrison L, McGinnis J, Ginsberg J. Low-dose oral vitamin K reliably reverses over-anticoagulation due to warfarin. *Thromb Haemost*. 1998;79:1116-1118.

18. Smirnov MD. Inhibition of activated protein C anticoagulant activity by prothrombin. *Blood*. 1999;94:3839-3846.

19. Abdelmalek MF, Spittell PC. 79-year-old woman with blue toes. *Mayo Clin Proc*. 1995;70:292-295.

20. Nagao T, Ibayashi S, Fujii K, Suimori H, Sadoshima S, Fujishima M. Treatment of warfarin-induced hair loss with ubidecarenone. *Lancet*. 1995;346:1104-1105. Letter.

21. Jamal SA, Browner WS, Bauer DC, Cummings SR. Warfarin use and risk for osteoporosis in elderly women. Study of Osteoporotic Fractures Research Group. *Ann Intern Med*. 1998;128:829-832.

22. Ginsburg JS. Use of antithrombotic agents during pregnancy. *Chest*. 1998;114:524S-530S.

23. Levine MN, Raskob G, Landefeld S, Kearon C. Hemorrhagic complications of anticoagulant treatment. *Chest*. 2001;119:108S-121S.

24. Hattersley PG, Mitsuoka JC, King JH. Sources of error in heparin therapy of thromboembolic disease. *Arch Intern Med*. 1980;140: 1173-1175.

25. Kitchens CS. Evaluation and treatment of bleeding associated with heparin and low-molecular-weight heparin administration. In: Alving BM, ed. *Blood components and Pharmacologic Agents in the Treatment of Congenital and Acquired Bleeding Disorders*. Bethesda Md: AABB Press; 2000:167-184.

26. Landefeld CS, Beyth RJ. Anticoagulant-related bleeding: clinical epidemiology, prediction, and prevention. *Am J Med*. 1993;95:315-328.

27. Nieuwenhuis HK, Albada J, Banga JD, Sixma JJ. Identification of risk factors for bleeding during treatment of acute venous thromboembolism with heparin or low molecular weight heparin. *Blood*. 1991;78:2337-2343.

28. Owens EL, Kasten GW, Hessel EA. Spinal subarachnoid hematoma after lumbar puncture and heparinization: a case report, review of the literature, and discussion of anesthetic implications. *Anesth Analg*. 1986;65:1201-1207.

29. Wysowski DK, Talarico L, Bacsanyi J, Botstein P. Spinal and epidural hematoma and low-molecular-weight heparin. *N Engl J Med*. 1998;338:1774-1775. Letter.

30. Horlocker TT, Heit JA. Low molecular weight heparin: biochemistry, pharmacology, perioperative prophylaxis regimens, and guidelines for regional anesthetic management. *Anesth Analg*. 1997;85: 874-885.

31. Wolzt M, Weltermann A, Nieszpaur-Los M, et al. Studies on the neutralizing effects of protamine on unfractionated and low molecular weight heparin (Fragmin) at the site of activation of the coagulation system in man. *Thromb Haemost*. 1995;73:439-443.

32. Warkentin TE, Chong BH, Greinacher A. Heparin-induced thrombocytopenia: towards consensus. *Thromb Haemost*. 1998;79:1-7.

33. Greinacher A, Potzsch B, Amiral J, Dummel V, Eichner A, Mueller-Eckhardt C. Heparin-associated thrombocytopenia: isolation of the antibody and characterization of a multimolecular PF4-heparin complex as the major antigen. *Thromb Haemost*. 1994;71:247-251.

34. Warkentin TE, Elavathil LJ, Hayward CP, Johnston MA, Russett JI, Kelton JG. The pathogenesis of venous limb gangrene associated with heparin-induced thrombocytopenia. *Ann Intern Med*. 1997;127:804-812.

35. Magnani HN. Heparin-induced thrombocytopenia (HIT): an overview of 230 patients treated with orgaran (ORG10172) [published correction appears *Thromb Haemost*. 1993;70:1072]. *Thromb Haemost*. 1993;70:554-561.

36. Warkentin TE, Kelton JG. Temporal aspects of heparin-induced thrombocytopenia. *N Engl J Med*. 2001;344:1286-1292.

18

37. Potzsch B, Klovekorn WP, Madlener K. Use of heparin during cardiopulmonary bypass in patients with a history of heparin-induced thrombocytopenia. *N Engl J Med*. 2000;343:515. Letter.

38. Muir JM, Hirsh J, Weitz JI, Andrew M, Young E, Shaughnessy SG. A histomorphometric comparison of the effects of heparin and low-molecular-weight heparin on cancellous bone in rats. *Blood*. 1997;89: 3236-3242.

39. Bhandari M, Hirsh J, Weitz JI, Young E, Venner TJ, Shaughnessy SG. The effects of standard and low molecular weight heparin on bone nodule formation in vitro. *Thromb Haemost*. 1998;80:413-417.

40. Walenga JM, Bick RL. Heparin-induced thrombocytopenia, paradoxical thromboembolism, and other side effects of heparin therapy. *Med Clin North Am*. 1998;82:635-658.

41. Bircher AJ, Itin PH, Buchner SA. Skin lesions, hypereosinophilia, and subcutaneous heparin. *Lancet*. 1994;343:861. Letter.

42. Majoor CL. Aldosterone suppression by heparin. *N Engl J Med*. 1968; 279:1172-1173.

43. Canova CR, Fischler MP, Reinhart WH. Effect of low-molecular-weight heparin on serum potassium. *Lancet*. 1997;349:1447-1448. Letter.

44. Anderson DR, Ginsberg JS, Burrows R, Brill-Edwards P. Subcutaneous heparin therapy during pregnancy: a need for concern at the time of delivery. *Thromb Haemost*. 1991;65:248-250.

45. Douketis JD, Ginsberg JS, Burrows RF, Duku EK, Webber CE, Brill-Edwards P. The effects of long-term heparin therapy during pregnancy on bone density. A prospective matched cohort study. *Thromb Haemost*. 1996;75:254-257.

46. Loscalzo J. Fibrinolytic therapy. In: Beutler E, Lichtman MA, Coller BS, eds. *Williams Hematology*. 5th ed. New York, NY: McGraw-Hill, Inc; 1994:1585-1591.

47. Gurwitz JH, Gore JM, Goldberg RJ, et al. Risk for intracranial hemorrhage after tissue plasminogen activator treatment for acute myocardial infarction. Participants in the National Register of Myocardial Infarction 2. *Ann Intern Med*. 1998;129:597-604.

48. Maggioni AP, Franzosi MG, Santoro E, White H, Van de Werf F, Tognoni G. The risk of stroke in patients with acute myocardial infarction after thrombolytic and antithrombotic treatment. Gruppo Italiano per lo Studio della Sopravvivenza nell 'Infarto Micardico II (GISSI-2), and the International Study Group. *New Engl J Med*. 1992;327:1-6.

49. Merlini PA, Ardissino D, Bauer KA, et al. Activation of the hemo-static mechanism during thrombolysis in patients with unstable an-gina pectoris. *Blood*. 1995;86:3327-3332.

50. Brenot F, Pacouret G, Meyer G, Sors H, Charbonnier B, Simonneau G. Adverse reactions with anistreplase. *Lancet*. 1991;338:114-115. Letter.

18

19

19

325

19

19

19

19

335

19

338

19

19

346

19

19

19

351